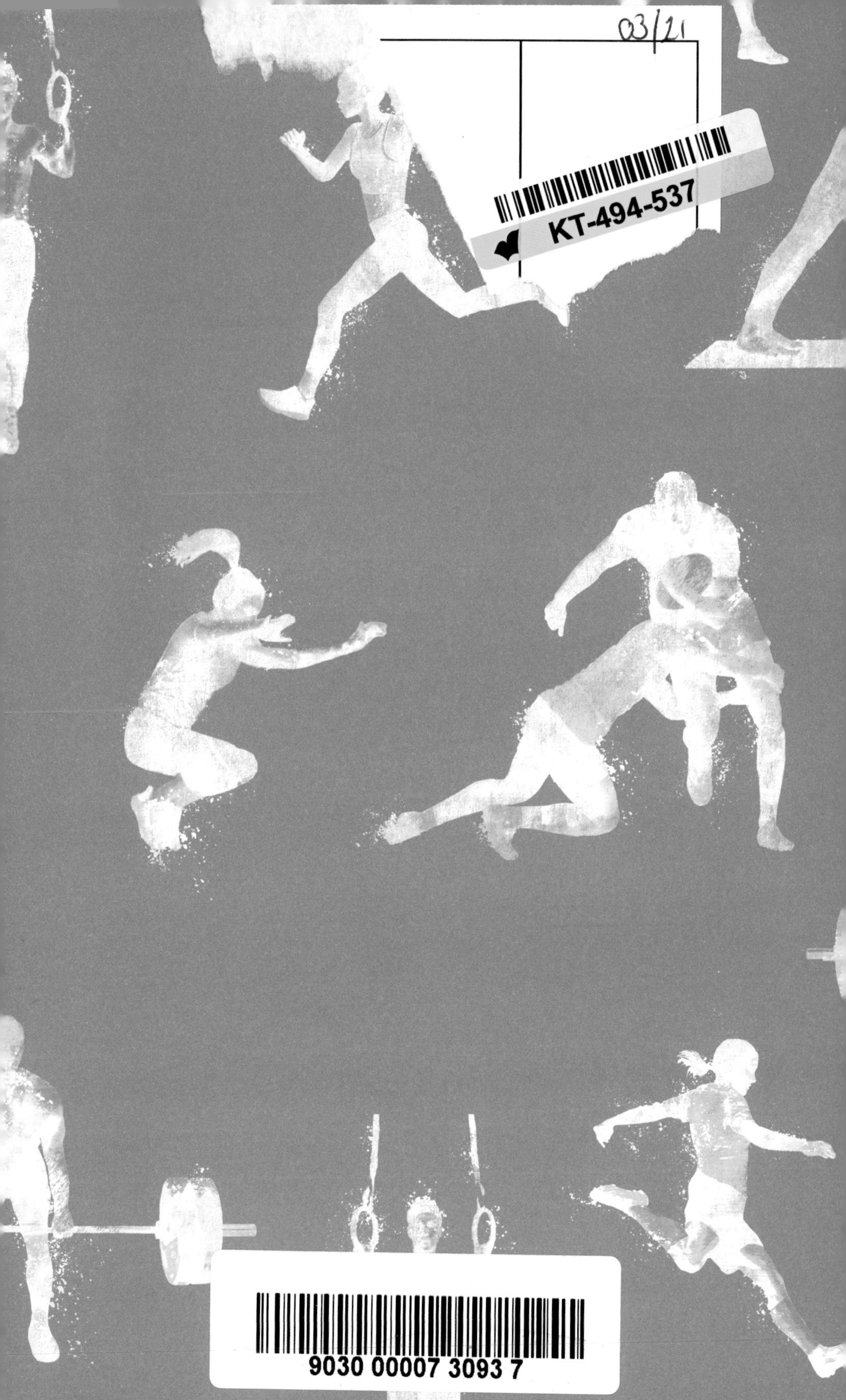

FIT

FIT

SMASH YOUR GOALS AND STAY STRONG FOR LIFE

Paul Olima

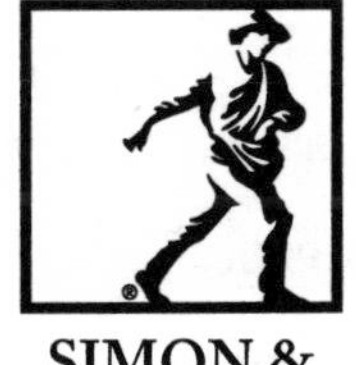

SIMON & SCHUSTER

London · New York · Sydney · Toronto · New Delhi

First published in Great Britain by Simon & Schuster UK Ltd, 2021

1 3 5 7 9 10 8 6 4 2

Simon & Schuster UK Ltd
1st Floor
222 Gray's Inn Road
London WC1X 8HB

www.simonandschuster.co.uk
www.simonandschuster.com.au
www.simonandschuster.co.in

Simon & Schuster Australia, Sydney
Simon & Schuster India, New Delhi

The author and publishers have made all reasonable efforts to contact copyright-holders for permission, and apologise for any omissions or errors in the form of credits given. Corrections may be made to future printings.

This book is not intended as a substitute for medical advice or treatment. It is recommended that readers always consult with a qualified medical practitioner or suitable therapist. While every effort has been made to verify the information provided, neither the author nor the publisher can accept responsibility for any errors or omissions that may be found in the text, or any actions taken by the reader as a result of reliance on the information contained in the text.

A CIP catalogue record for this book is available from the British Library

Hardback ISBN: 978-1-4711-9750-5
Trade Paperback ISBN: 978-1-4711-9751-2
eBook ISBN: 978-1-4711-9752-9

Typeset in Bembo by M Rules

Printed in the UK by CPI Group (UK) Ltd, Croydon, CR0 4YY

I'd like to dedicate this book to my two wonderful daughters who mean the world to me, Caramel Zeus and Baby Zeus. You have both given my life more meaning and made me feel complete as a human. Love you more than anything – your dad, Black Zeus.

CONTENTS

PART 4 YOUR WHOLE-BODY HEALTH

INTRODUCTION

Howareya, I'm Paul, aka Black Zeus: a personal trainer, meathead, gym lover, fitness freak, former footballer and rugby player, dad to two girls, London-living, Irish-speaking Black lad, made in Dublin by way of Nigeria.

I've written this book because I believe fitness will change your life for the better. Your body is a powerhouse created to protect you, and you owe it to yourself to move it. It's the only one you've got and most bits don't grow back, so let's take care of it. I've spent nearly two decades playing professional and semi-professional sport, and training at a high level, in addition to being a PT and qualified football coach. I've picked up a lot of knowledge along the way on fitness, regimens and the lifestyle habits needed to support intensive training. And I also know what's utter crap. I can speak from experience about the pitfalls of training without really knowing what you're doing – that was once me.

Fitness isn't about flashy gyms, it's not about looking a certain way, weighing yourself daily or keeping up with the latest daft exercise trends. You don't need to have an all-or-nothing approach – it's not just about suddenly signing up for an Ironman to enjoy the day-to-day benefits of fitness. Making little steps towards wellness is every bit as valuable. You might never have set foot in a gym, never have jogged or played a sport, to be enjoying peak performance. It's about being active while doing something you love: playing frisbee in the park with friends, dancing with your kids in the kitchen, swimming in the warm sea on holiday. And it can be deceptive too – I'm on the front cover of this book half-naked (and, okay, being a bit of a poser), but it might surprise you that my type of 'fit' means I can barely run for a bus, much less any distance longer, because I am seriously lacking in *aerobic* fitness (i.e. the type of fitness that generates oxygen, transferring it around the body). This doesn't mean I'm unhealthy, it's just that I choose to put my main focus into weightlifting, and any cardio I do will detract from my lifting gains.

Health and fitness underpin our entire wellbeing and, frankly, I don't give a rat's if you're roller skating, curling or playing Muggle Quidditch – I just want you to move. Your body is a beautiful thing. You may not think that right now, but once you read about what's going on behind the scenes to keep you alive, I think you'll learn to have a profound respect for it. And knowing that you can feel and look better every single day, as well as prolonging your life, all by sitting down a bit less, is a no-brainer. The body is designed to move – it's begging you to, to help future-proof your health.

The mental benefits are every bit as (or even more) important – exercise can make you more focused, less stressed and more resilient to what life has to throw at you. Harvard psychiatry professor John Ratey says it even rivals prescription anti-depressants like Prozac for its mood-boosting qualities, particularly when done at a level that burns around 1,600 calories a week. It's why GPs now often 'prescribe' exercise, as part of a wider plan, for patients suffering low mood. I can definitely vouch for it affecting my frame of mind – I'm satanic if something gets in the way of me exercising.

If you are new to fitness or trying to get back into it after a pause, we'll get to the root of what's been holding you back and wave bye-bye to any PE PTSD that might be lingering. Getting out there is nothing to be afraid of. In fact, it's the opposite: it's the gift that keeps on giving, making you feel good inside and out. If you've picked this book up thinking that you hate exercise but do it begrudgingly, then you just haven't found your *thing* yet. There is a form of exercise out there that you will love, and by the end of the book you'll have found it. And if you're already a certified training maniac, I will show you how to achieve even greater things than you thought possible. Understanding the science of what's happening inside your body every time you move means you can harness it to get the specific results you're looking for, to smash beyond a plateau, beat any obstacle and boost your performance, whatever your level.

There are carefully devised workouts in the book, from gym-based weightlifting to plyometrics and yoga, to cardio-based sports like running, put together by me along with some insights from some of the world's top experts in those areas. At different times of my life I've tried them all. There's no 'perfect' exercise, no one-size-fits-all, but by finding something you actually like, it will feel like a challenge rather than a chore. The plans I give all have one thing in common: they will get you moving. You might be someone who is HIIT-mad and only wants to focus on that, or you might like to see these as a pick 'n' mix, alternating between several to keep things varied. It's all good! We're all different and our needs and goals vary depending on factors such as our current condition, age and what we like doing. Similarly, how we respond to exercise will be slightly different.

We'll also be talking nutrition, lifestyle and how to harness the mentality of a top athlete to ensure you achieve your health goals, whether that's feeling more energised, getting stronger, trimming down or building muscle mass to make you more powerful.

Benefits of exercise

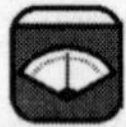 · Aids healthy weight management

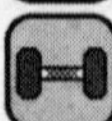 · Improves strength

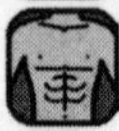 · Tones the body by causing fat-loss and muscle gain

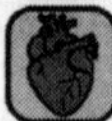 · Protects organs from becoming fatty

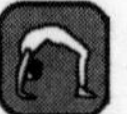 · Improves flexibility

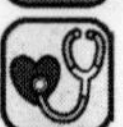 · Helps prevent diseases such as type 2 diabetes and hypertension

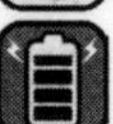 · Increases energy and stops you feeling so tired

 · Lowers stress

 · Improves sleep

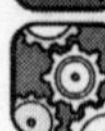 · Makes you feel sharper, more focused and more productive

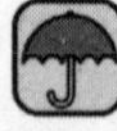 · Gives you more resilience so you're better able to cope with life's curveballs

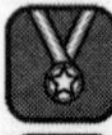 · Boosts confidence and self-belief

 · Makes you feel better in yourself generally

 · Gives you a more positive outlook and opens you up to new opportunities

The life and times of Black Zeus

Firstly, let me introduce you to my alter ego: Black Zeus. If you're familiar with Greek mythology, you'll know that Zeus was the chief Olympian god, of the sky and thunder. Sounds a bit grand for a tracksuit-wearing north Dubliner (living in south London) to be comparing himself to Zeus, but hold on – don't bin the book just yet! – let me explain. There are many things I admire about the fella. For one, he tried to keep everyone happy by being fair. Also, he was carefree and made a point of laughing a lot. For Zeus, the success of others made him happy, not envious. And these are traits that I aspire to. Okay, Zeus was a bit of a rogue, what with his occasional spot of kidnapping and cannibalism, but I'll aim to draw the line there.

And who the hell am I to be telling you what to do, I hear you ask? A fair question. I have been a PT for ten years and, before then, since my teens, I've played football and rugby to professional and semi-professional levels. I'm also a powerbuilder (a combo of powerlifting and bodybuilding), so spend most days in the gym building my strength and shifting tin.

I had my first taste of the gym aged fourteen, when my friends and I would sneak into our local one in Dublin. I was naturally lean and I wanted to put some meat on the bones. After a few weeks of lifting weights I noticed my biceps getting bigger. There was something kind of magical about putting in the work and seeing results fairly quickly. I was soon hooked and the iron jungle has been my second home ever since. For the best part of a decade I combined strength training with cardio. I've done so many types of sports in my quest for fitness, I've pushed them all at some stage.

I grew up in Dublin, the second youngest (and prettiest) of six sports-obsessed boys who were all tough as old boots. All of us were named after saints, although I'm afraid we didn't tend to live up to the virtuous behaviour of our biblical namesakes! There was never a dull moment at home; it was always go-go-go. My dad had arrived in Ireland from Nigeria in the 1970s to study medicine and Mumsy followed afterwards with my oldest brother in tow. We lived in a lively Dublin suburb with loads of open green space and a little forest on our doorstep – almost all my memories revolve around being outside, running, playing football with all the neighbourhood kids. It was a brilliant community, where my dad was the local GP and we were easily spotted as 'the six Olima lads'. Mama Zeus started an IT business, which really took off. It was a time when many women would have been stay-at-home mums, especially as there were so many of us kids to look after, but she is so entrepreneurial. She's been a massive inspiration to me on that front. Both my auld fella and lady would always tell us that hard work was the key to success (I'd often get this ear-bashing when I was playing video games instead of doing my homework).

Strong values were drilled into me as a kid and became even more engrained playing sports.

Ever since school, I've always tried to bring people up with me. I wouldn't stand by watching someone be bullied – that cool-kid hierarchy was so far away from what I felt. I always made an effort to watch out for the smaller guy in the class, or the quieter, more shy one. I think that must be part of the reason I became a trainer – I want everyone to feel included, to help build people up (especially when arseholes were trying to take them down) so that we all feel empowered, like we can take on the world together. It makes us better humans.

I try to apply this to all of my work, including one of my jobs, which is sports choreography – helping directors behind the scenes on ad sets instruct the star how to move. I'm often hired for campaigns with footballers, rugby players and boxers, where my role is to interpret what the director or photographer wants and then communicate that to the athletes, suggesting specific moves. Filming might be done in a small studio or sometimes on location – for example, I flew out to South Africa with Nike to film the South African international women's football team and was also being part of the crew for the British Lions tour adverts. This is the best job – it's so much fun.

If I can't have fun working, I don't want to do it. Life is far too short. I kind of see myself as a professional fluffer – trying to give energy, warming people up so that they can go off and do great things. This is essential for PTs everywhere. They are there to motivate and help facilitate others; it should never be about them or their egos.

Now's the time

There are more gyms and personal trainers in business than ever before; it's a multi-billion-pound industry where, in the UK, having a membership to a gym or to fitness classes is as common as having a supermarket points card.

Before we start, however, I want you to forget what you think you know about training and fitness. There are so many misconceptions about fitness and training that make it seem like it's harder than it really is.

I want to cut through the fitness industry's bollocks, because there's a lot of misinformation out there – including from brands and leading fitness personalities who are deliberately misleading us, making people think that fitness is much more complicated than it is. But it's not a mystery; it's basic physiology – and your radar for bullshit will be state-of-the-art after reading this book. Is it any wonder we're all confused, when we're being bombarded with contradictory messages? There are a lot of convincing cowboys out there and it's no surprise many have amassed a substantial social media following. Glossy hair and glowing teeth, they make it look so easy. Some of these mega-reach influencers don't even have a basic PT qualification but are posting exercises that thousands – sometimes millions – of fans are copying at home or in the gym. Thing is, though – I've seen some of these influencers do shitty clickbait exercise videos for the 'Gram, then do their own hardcore session afterwards, which is the reason they look like they do, though their feed would have you think it's by doing a gentle pull of a resistance band.

I started parodying some of these videos on Insta, mainly so that I could dress up in a blonde wig and play a background soundtrack of kazoo (a beautiful, much-overlooked instrument). I've come under some flak from keyboard warriors for doing so, but I've found it's the people who know what they're doing the least who love getting offended the most. I don't discriminate – whether it's a pal or a favourite fit-girl influencer, I'll be having a laugh at both. And I'd expect the very same from them, were I to do a ropey instructive video. Bring it on! If you're putting yourself out there on social media and earning a nice living from it, you need to grow a thick skin and be prepared for people not to tolerate shit advice.

These homework videos really came into their own during lockdown. Honestly, I'm suffering flashbacks from the horror show of some – people using toilet roll as resistance, strange prancing in leotards, some even embroiling their poor defensive pets (who look mortified, tainted by association) in their living room routines. If you didn't laugh, you'd cry (sometimes I do).

So, if you're reading this and putting out dodgy reels with no science behind the moves along with WTF form, get ready, because I'll be slapping you with the back of my glove and telling you to wise up. I'm speaking out not because I'm a hater, but the opposite! I love fitness and want everyone to respect it, finding something that works for them. When I was six years old and painting a banging picture at school, my classmate Sharon came over to me and sighed: 'Paul, your picture is great. Mine is really bad,' clearly looking for sympathy. I looked from her artwork into her soft doe-eyes and said, 'Yes, Sharon, your picture's shite.' Cue tears, a bollocking from the teacher, who then ratted me out to my mum. But, Shazza, what if you'd grown up with everyone pandering to you, telling you you were the next Tracey Emin, only for you to find out in adulthood when someone finally had the temerity to set you straight? Mate, I did you a favour, and I'm applying this logic to all the fitness darlings out there.

The problem is that people follow these shit workouts and they don't end up looking like Kim Kardashian (you know, from that picture that broke the internet), so they think it's something *they've* done wrong. It can put people off for life, affecting their entire wellbeing for the worse. So, what I want to do is set you straight. I've made many (seriously – loads) of training mistakes in the past, wasted my time doing pointless regimes that over-promised and under-delivered. I've thrown my cash away on supplements that did sweet FA. And then there were the things I didn't to do which I should have, such as properly preparing my body for training by mobilising correctly and taking time to recover from injury. Basically, I've seen it all and I know what will get results and what to sack off. And I'm also aware how mental blocks can sometimes make putting a pair of trainers on feel like a hike up Everest.

How to navigate this book

This is a book to help you on whatever stage of the fitness journey you're on. If the thought of lashing on a pair of leggings and trainers is intimidating enough, I will hold your hand (not literally – I'm writing this book during the pandemic, so am keeping 2m apart from humans at all times). Or you might be a habitual goer, plodding along to the gym a couple of times a week but only doing semi-effective workouts – I will show you how to breathe new life into your fitness routine and make the time you spend on it so much more useful. If you are an accomplished athlete who wants to reach peak power, I will get you to the next level. By the time you finish this book, you'll have acquired the same know-how as a Level 2 personal trainer or fitness instructor.

Whether you're looking for practical advice, motivation or inspiration, there's something here for you. The first part of the book taps into mindset, and this might be particularly relevant if you have struggled in the past to motivate yourself to exercise or if you have fallen off the wagon. Identifying any blocks from the start, and exploring them, will really help you stay steadfast on this quest. When you're honest with yourself, you become more committed and you get *better* results. This book teaches you ways to be accountable to yourself and to your goals; your determination will grow as you quickly start noticing the results of your workouts.

I want you to come away bursting with energy to start or go back to fitness, to get much more from what you're doing now by working out smarter. Whatever you goal is, we'll make it happen – and even if you're currently unsure of what your goal should be, we'll look into how to set one. You'll gain an understanding of what hasn't worked in the past and have a toolkit to fill in any gaps in your knowledge of how your body works, the role of sleep and diet, and what different forms of exercise offer. Think of this book as having a PT – but without forking out vast sums of cash. The way I work as a trainer, reaching clients through my online programmes, is that people sign up as a one-off. The same goes for this book – my guidance lays the foundations for your training success in the future. You learn it once and then you don't need to keep coming back for more hand-holding – you will have the expertise to direct your own training, even when your goals evolve. The information is this book is targeted to all sexes and age groups, as well as all levels of experience.

You'll be getting workout plans on a range of sports, which are suitable for all levels, along with practical advice on getting started and excelling, in addition to real-life expertise from some of the fittest people in the world. I could write a whole book on any one of the exercises covered, there's so much to say about them all. So, what you have here is a decent overview of how and why they work and a brilliant plan for all levels that you can start today. I've written each of these plans and called in some words of wisdom from some serious bosses who are experts in that particular sport. I've also tried and tested each of these workouts myself, so they have the Black Zeus seal of approval. Many of the movements and exercises described in Part 3 of the book are demonstrated in short videos on my website www.theomegaarmy.com/workout-videos.

While I give you workouts, I am also wary of being overly prescriptive. Learning to tune into your body, in order to understand when it needs to be pushed and when it needs to chill, will be far more useful than stumping up your hard-earned coinage on a trainer month in, month out, telling you exactly what to do. In the short term, PTs can be a brilliant way of motivating you and helping to get you started, but see it as a dirty fling rather than a marriage.

I'm going to be giving you a bit of tough love too, because I know you can handle it. I won't take any prisoners. If you're easily offended, put the book down now, because this is a snowflake-free zone! But if you stick with me, you will achieve amazing things.

PART 1

WHAT'S STOPPING YOU?

IT'S GO-TIME

Roll up, roll up, it's time to get started, folks. If you're gearing yourself up for your very first trip to the gym or beginning a brand new regime after you've been stuck in a training rut, let's free the athlete within (and it *is* in there, dormant – I'm telling you – even if it's currently sharing a home in your gut with some salty snacks).

This section is all about working out what you want to achieve, and bringing body and mind together to make it happen through setting smart goals. We'll be harnessing your inner strength for outer power, laying the groundwork for the physical work that follows in the next section. I'll be drawing on some popular theories too, devised by thinkers far brainier than myself, about the secrets to growing confidence, grit and success.

I speak from experience when I say there is no workout harder than getting your mind in gear, ready to take positive action in your life towards better health and wellbeing. The deadlift I do at the gym every week is a doddle by comparison! You will become an unstoppable force of nature, all by doing it your way. When you find an activity you love, your body will love doing it too. It doesn't take a genius to know that the mind and body are intrinsically linked, so boosting one will boost the other. There's an emerging trend for fitness that targets both the body and mind; there are even mental health gyms cropping up, helping people tap into what they want to achieve, thereby making the most out of their sessions. Having a mind–body connection will not just support good mental health, motivating you to exercise in the first place – it'll maximise your performance when you do.

> 'I was extremely shy as a kid, to the point my parents thought there was something wrong with me. It wasn't until they watched me playing sports they realised that was the way I expressed myself, becoming a leader on the pitch. Sports became an outlet for me, a way of coming out of my comfort zone.'
>
> EMILE HESKEY, FORMER ENGLAND AND LIVERPOOL FOOTBALLER

To me, there are four pillars of fitness, and you'll notice that I come back to these time and time again, because they underpin our whole health – body and mind.

1. Athleticism

This is the pinnacle of fitness – if you are training, whether a beginner or elite athlete, you'll soon find that energy, agility and endurance are key to your success, whatever your exercise of choice. And the good news is that you don't need to be a born athlete to excel. That myth has been doing the rounds for too long and sometimes (and understandably so) holds people back. You might think, for example, *What's the point in dusting off the bike? I'm not built like Victoria Pendleton, so I'm going to stay within my comfort zone.* But if you work hard, it'll pay dividends.

2. Strength

This manifests itself differently depending on the training you're doing. Whether it's the strength that comes from lifting weights or from cardiovascular training, it's a fundamental foundation of fitness. Clients often come to me saying they want to follow a regime that will make them look a certain way, but I always tell them to start by building strength and that will lead to aesthetic changes. It's often the case that while weight loss is their initial goal, in the end it's the fact that they *feel* so much better that gets them hooked.

3. Diversity

If you get anything out of reading this book (and you bleedin' better), it should be finding your 'thing'. Even if you were the chubby kid at school, or the gangliest one in the class with two left feet and the last to be picked for games, I promise you there is a form of exercise out there that you'll enjoy. So throw away any memories of inadequacy, because I'll help you find your thing if you haven't already. Success (whatever that looks like for you) will be far more likely when you find something you like doing, be it CrossFit or trampolining.

Similarly, if you have been put off by the depiction of the wellness industry as being dominated by long, blonde Aphrodites wearing £100 leggings, then take heart in the fact that it seems to be gradually becoming more diverse. Thank feck. That exclusive, elitist clique is the antithesis of true sport. If that's making you feel like an outsider, look towards our incredible professional athletes, Olympians and Paralympians who represent true diversity and who are an inspiration of strength and power. Don't be looking to Johnny-what's-his-chops on Instagram, oiled up with his orange fake tan and little-sister shorts – there's no inspiration to be found there.

4. Confidence

There's not a lot in life that isn't affected by confidence. It will unlock your potential, propelling you forwards with a tenacity that allows you to achieve your goals. And lacking it will do the opposite. You might be lucky enough to have been born with buckets of confidence or had an amazing family who instilled it in you and nurtured it from a young age. Or maybe it hasn't been quite so rosy and confidence is a skill you need some help adopting. Mental strength underpins everything, and it's absolutely something that can be learned. It's by far the most important pillar, and it's why I'll be banging on about it throughout the book.

Unleash your power

I'll be bandying about the terms 'fitness', 'health' and 'strength', but in reality it's not always easy to define these, as they mean different things to different people. Am I fit? Yes, I can lift small donkey (I can but I don't!), but I'd be completely knackered jogging a 5k. On the other hand, the Kenyan marathon record-holder Eliud Kipchoge can zip around 26.2 miles in just under two hours, but I can't imagine his bench-pressing is up to much. He and I are both 'fit', because fitness comes in different guises.

I'm also not saying my passion, which is lifting weights,

combining powerlifting and bodybuilding (powerbuilding, if you will), is the best thing you can do to build overall fitness. It's not. Ensuring my body can lift a few hundred kilos at one time means that my rigorous conditioning programme would be damaged if I did another type of exercise, like more cardio. So, some people would look at me and think my type of fitness is skewed in one direction, that I'm not an all-rounder – and they'd be right. (And that includes my mum, who doesn't like me lifting heavy weights and still laments my naturally lean frame, last seen in the late '90s!) If you want to work to an elite level, there comes a point where you've got to give the discipline of your choice no less than 100%, because throwing anything else into the mix will make you less good at it. If you've ever watched something like the World's Strongest Man or Woman competitions on TV, you'll see the extreme lengths that these athletes go to in order to be on top of their game. Eyes bulging, noses bleeding, veins popping – it's the Wild West of sports. They are totally and completely dedicated; nothing comes before the sport for them – not even family. At that level, to be the best, you have got to want it so much that everything else in life takes a backseat.

When I think about what makes me feel healthy, it comes down to energy and strength. Having the energy to keep up with my kids, lug the two of them (and their infinite kit) around, kick a ball about in the park. It's being able to do tasks efficiently and with strength, without discomfort. So, yes, you can absolutely be fit up to a level that won't have Ellie Simmonds quaking in her togs. And what I come back to time and time again is that this isn't about looking a certain way – it's about your body having the power and energy within it to achieve the tasks you want it to. That might be bouldering, Pilates or salsa dancing. And when you challenge your body and condition it, it will naturally affect what you see on the outside, but to me that's not the priority.

The pitch, the ball and me

I know first-hand the importance of finding something in life you're passionate about – both in fitness and in all other parts of life. As a kid, football was my be-all and end-all. I was naturally sporty from the get-go and I never had any trouble making friends because I was always around to kick a ball about, and football was everything to the local kids in the suburb of Dublin where I grew up. I had a reputation really early on for being 'the Black lad who's deadly at football'. If you were on my team, you'd be winning! As a teenager, I played for the top Dublin youth teams, putting way more energy into training and matches than I did into school lessons and homework.

When I'd finished school and was about to start a course at a local college (electronic engineering, which was very much not my life-long dream), I got a call to see if I wanted to try out for West Ham. Er . . . getting paid to play football? *Yes, please.* So I packed my trunk and off to the UK I went.

I was raring to go, really believing I was on the edge of something massive. But the trial for West Ham was a disaster. So, I was temporarily transferred to Scunthorpe United and was there for four weeks. I was nailing it in the training, and we were building up to play against Sheffield United; it was going really well. But when the day of the match came, again I didn't perform well. I had been running every day to make sure I was super-fit, so that nothing would get in the way of playing for Scunthorpe; I was fit as a fiddle. But when we played that match against Sheffield United, I had my hands on my hips, gasping, in the first five minutes. I could barely last the first half; I couldn't even breathe. I had been training hard, but not training smart, and at that stage, when I was only nineteen, I didn't know enough about the body to figure out what was going wrong and what I really needed to do to progress.

Scunthorpe told me I needed to get match-fit before they'd consider signing me. It was pretty disappointing; I'd built up a great vibe with the coaches and players, feeling part of the team. While they recognised I had the talent, they highlighted how lacking I was in endurance. From there I went to Bristol Rovers and began a few years of hopping from team to team, waiting for a big break that would get me spotted. I was living in a flatshare in Bristol with four lads and working my (football) socks off, now playing for Taunton Town, trying to raise my fitness so that I could return to Bristol Rovers. When I turned up to Bristol's stadium expecting to trial in a pre-season friendly against Swansea, it turned out the manager hadn't confirmed my trial and instead there was some Rickie Lambert fella on the pitch, playing in my position. And, as it turns out, Rickie's career took him from Bristol Rovers to Liverpool FC (to add insult to injury, they're the team I've supported since I was in short trousers). He went on to play international football too, being capped many times for England. Had I played that day as I was meant to, would I have been heading off to the Premier League? Rickie Lambert, did you steal my career?!

Who knows how it might have panned out that day if I had

trialled. Maybe I'd be living it up in a Merseyside mansion, making cameos on *The Real Housewives of Cheshire*. One can only dream. Anyway, I figured I had been dropped by Bristol. My agent hadn't even bothered to tell me. I started questioning whether football was for me. I really believed that if you wanted something enough it would happen, but it just wasn't coming together. Looking back, though, I can see now that this wasn't the course I was meant to take.

I got invited to play for Dagenham & Redbridge, who had just been promoted into the League from the Conference. I was in the reserve squad and travelling from London to Dagenham every day, taking two tubes or driving the A406 for over two hours I stayed for two years playing reserve football, never quite able to break through to the first team. While there, they put me out on loan to the semi-pro leagues and, again, it just felt like I was treading water, in some kind of limbo, waiting for something big to happen. Having felt on the cusp of achieving a career in top-tier football, it felt as though that dream was slipping through my fingers. And I was fed up. It occurred to me that maybe football just wasn't my thing; maybe this wasn't meant to be. That's a pretty hard realisation to come to when, for so many years, since being a kid scoring all the goals for my local teams in Dublin, I had envisioned a future playing with the pros. I'll admit, I wallowed a bit . . . Where had it gone wrong? Could I have trained even harder, made better decisions, had better expert advice? Probably. Scunthorpe was the point it could have gone either way – maybe if I'd been better prepared fitness-wise, it could have been a stepping stone to the Premier League. Who knows?

When I left Dagenham & Redbridge, I ended up signing

with Grays Athletic, a team in the league below. They were a professional outfit in that they trained every day, and it was good to be part of their first team for once, as previously I had always been with the reserves, which was frustrating to say the least. So I felt happy to be on the front line, being part of the team and wearing the kit with pride. I've noticed that there's a bit of a trend now for young players who'd prefer to play for the reserves of a Premier League team than for the firsts of a second-tier team. I would totally challenge this ethos as, having done both, I can say for sure that playing for the first team – even if it is for a less prestigious club – is so much more motivating.

I'd played a season at Grays, all the while still being obsessed with watching football on TV. Whoever was playing and whatever league, I'd be glued to the screen, analysing every move, trying to work out the strategy, thinking about what I'd do differently were I the trainer. I just loved it. I decided to get a coaching qualification with the view to someday being a professional coach, so I studied to get my FA level 2 coaching badge. Around this time I moved down another league to play for Thurrock. Just like getting my football coaching qualifications, I decided to diversify my skills more and started earning my fitness instructor qualifications. I felt like this made sense, given my passion for fitness as well as being naturally sociable and upbeat, so I was keen to combine these to help people get in shape. I loved studying to be a PT. I was in my element learning about how the body works, what happens to it during exercise, the amazing ability it has to adapt and get stronger. It was pretty different from school, where I couldn't care less about finding pi or identifying v-shaped valleys. I'd been banging the gym for about seven years by this point and seeing good enough results, but doing this course was a game-changer for me. Suddenly I was learning about the science behind what was happening to me and how the different factors all came together in a jigsaw. It was heaven. I dived in and was immediately hooked.

Around this time I got a job at a gym in London as a fitness instructor. So, at this point I was earning my keep playing semi-pro football in Essex and being a personal trainer/fitness instructor at the gym two hours away in west London. I was on the road a lot over those three years.

At this stage I'd also started on the next round of study for football coaching, doing the UEFA B course, and I started thinking that while I absolutely love the beautiful game, I maybe didn't want to be a full-time coach. I asked myself what I loved and told myself to focus on that, job-wise – so strength and conditioning was the way forward. I played for a few more teams after Thurrock (I had more clubs than Tiger Woods), but it became clear in my mind that the body was where it was at for me. I had almost finished my UEFA B course when I dropped out and put my energy into a strength and conditioning learning course. It made me rethink football too. Football had been my life for so many years, but the more I learned about the body and how it could be conditioned, the more I wanted to move away from football training with its focus on cardio, primarily through running. I was tired. Tired of running endlessly. Tired of the long commutes to training. I wanted a new challenge, to redirect my fitness and put my body through its paces to see how strong and powerful I could become.

I left semi-pro football and it felt like the right decision. I'd lost the love for it, and I felt a bit battered from being passed from club to club just to try to earn a living. I had given everything I could by that point, and in life sometimes you need to learn when to walk away. I am a big believer that as soon as one door closes, another opens – you just need to be willing to see opportunities when they come your way.

Stop saying 'tomorrow'

> 'Many a false step is made by standing still.'
>
> CHINESE PROVERB

If exercise is something you've been meaning to do but keep putting off, it's time to seize the day. Years from now, you're far more likely to regret the things you *didn't* do than the things you did. It's often a heartache for those unable to move like they used to – whether through older age or maybe being less mobile through illness – that they wish they could move more. So, what's stopping you today? Here are the most common excuses I hear (and I give some of my solutions for them a little further on):

It's too late to start, I've haven't exercised before and it hasn't done me any harm

Sorry to break it to you, but you probably have been causing damage to yourself unknowingly, and starting now can help reverse that. It's never too late; whether you're 5 or 105, you will benefit, physically and mentally, from even a small amount of exercise, so don't let age be your excuse. And remember, if you have kids, you will be setting them an amazing example by embracing exercise, teaching them it's an essential part of life.

Exercise is boring

Your cousin Sunita swears by spin, she's been going for months and is radiating health. You tried it and loathed every minute – the bright flashing lights, rave music and hyperactive instructor make you want to scream into your sweat-soaked headband. So, don't go back! Find something else, because there's no one-size-fits-all. We are unique beings; one person's hell is another's heaven. For me, heaven is the sound of clinking iron in a gloomy, stinking, cave-like lifters' gym, but I have no doubt that that would have many running for the hills, especially if you're an outdoorsy type (in which case you might literally be running for the hills).

I know nothing about the latest fitness trends

Fuck that. Those who take their dog for a good brisk walk every day, week in, week out, come rain or shine, will likely be among the fittest people you know. Are they doing HulaFit? Mate, they have no clue what that is. And they don't need to!

Sports and gyms are just for the super-athletic, not for the likes of me

As someone who has a naturally lean frame, I remember sneaking into gyms as a teenager, in awe of the stacked bodies

I was seeing, mine being more of the weedy variety. And I know what it's like to walk into a room and feel like you stand out – during my childhood this was usually the case because of my skin colour. It's not always easy, and if you're someone who feels uncomfortable even wearing the kit, try to remember that people are focusing on their own shit and not looking at you. Starting is the hardest part and it gets easier each time you do it.

Exercise is just another thing to feel guilty about when you can't do it

Life does sometimes get in the way and you won't be able to make every session, whether that's due to other commitments or because you're just not in the mood. It's important to listen to your body, and there's a subtle difference between not feeling *able* to exercise and not being arsed to. If you're finding one day that you want to work out but you're having to drag your sorry self off the sofa, just get into your kit and do two minutes of your workout. If you're still not feeling it, sack it off that day – it's not meant to be.

I'm only exercising to lose weight but I'm not seeing any results

No, no, no, no – weight loss should *not* be your key motivator! Your weight is one part of a much bigger health picture. Stop obsessing over your reflection; when you *feel* good, you'll *look* good.

IT'S ALL IN YOUR HEAD

You don't have to be born with the physique of Nicola Adams or Usain Bolt to achieve amazing things in your sport of choice. Harnessing your mental strength can massively impact on your success – this kind of outlook is at the root of the athlete mentality at the gym. I know I'm sounding a bit Mystic Meg, but stay with me here. By setting yourself challenges and having a sense of focus, your overall determination will increase. It means that you will be more committed to succeed and not get derailed if a setback occurs.

The psychology around success is so important that it plays a vital role in every professional sport. Expert therapists work alongside athletes and teams to ensure their minds work in tandem with their bodies – that what's in their heads boosts their performance rather than impedes it. You will find it harder to succeed with your physical goals if your head isn't in the right place. You mightn't even be able to get off the couch, let alone into the gym. This is where outlook is everything, and fortunately, even if you are a born pessimist, and this has held you back in the past from exercising effectively, you can adapt your thinking.

You're going to have to check yourself here – ask yourself some questions and be brutally honest in your answers. A good place to start is by considering if you're someone with a *growth* or a *fixed* mindset. According to Carol Dweck, an expert in what motivates people, there are two ways of looking at life: if you have a fixed mindset, you might give up easily, avoid challenges, be unwilling to accept feedback that is less than complimentary and feel threatened by the success of others. So you can imagine that having a fixed mindset is kryptonite for anyone trying to motivate themselves when it comes to exercise. This way of looking at the world holds you back because it limits your ambition and stops you in your tracks before you even try. It makes you question what you've done in the past and blame yourself when things haven't gone to plan, rather than acknowledging that we are all human, we're a work in progress, and we won't get it right all the time - *boom! Move on!* It'll keep you in your comfort zone, so when you apply that to fitness, you might think, *Well, that training regime sounds too hard, I'll probably start but then drop out like I did the time before.* What you have done in the past does not define you; if it did, I'd still be ruminating about those nights at Inferno's nightclub where I may, once or twice, have ended up . . . No, I never think about that. Never. *Ever.* (I still kind of love Inferno's, though.)

On the other hand, if you have a growth mindset you embrace challenges and are tenacious in the face of setbacks; you learn from constructive criticism and you are inspired by the success of others, rather than it making you feel inadequate. The benefit of a growth mindset is that you feel you can make your own luck, that if you work hard, you will achieve. It's not about naturally being the cleverest, fittest or happiest person in the world (you're none of those things – #sorrynotsorry!), it's about feeling confident enough in yourself to go for it. It's empowering because it relies on you, and you alone, to get to where you want to be; it's not about needing validation from others or leaving it up to the gods to decide your fate.

You may naturally be someone who looks on the bright side and who isn't overly hampered by self-doubt, or you may be someone who needs to develop this more glass-half-full way of thinking. I think I fall into the former camp, and that may have been something that was shaped by my upbringing. Growing up in Dublin in the '90s was seriously mono-cultural; we were the only Black family around. We looked pretty different to other Irish people – who aren't exactly known for their dark complexions! I don't think I met another Black person there, outside of the family, until I was well into my teens. So, I was very used to walking into a classroom, football club, shop – wherever – and people noticing me.

Having said that, it never felt like a burden; it was the opposite – it felt like a superpower! I'm a natural extrovert, so I probably enjoyed standing out from the crowd. My main aim in life was to have fun. I had a great childhood and an amazing motley crew of friends. I was very outgoing and boisterous. There was an undercurrent of racism in Ireland, though, a tension bubbling below the surface, which sometimes boiled over. When I was six, my dad told me that if anyone called me the N-word, I could swing for them – and this licence to fight stayed with me! As I got older, the word would usually come out of someone's mouth just before or just after they received my fist in their face. I could certainly hold my own, as could most people in the area where I lived, and I had four older brothers after all! It was a fairly tough area where I grew up, so you learned to fight and it was sink or swim. These fisticuffs were a fairly regular occurrence, but I never really took the racist abuse to heart. I don't think it really fazed me because I always felt confident enough in myself to know it was just them being idiots. Anyway, my friends wouldn't have stood for me getting abused; with any hint of a racial slur, they were in like a flash throwing a punch, often before I could. As much as the shade of my skin set me apart in some ways, as a kid in Dublin, it also helped break down barriers. I was always the class clown, and having a laugh with classmates brought smiles all round. I think sharing jokes and messing about made everyone realise I was just like them. For a lot of these kids, I must have been the first non-white person they'd ever met.

I was amazed, when I moved to London fifteen years ago, at how little I stood out! Whereas in Dublin the colour of my skin made me a bit of a novelty, in London it was nothing of the sort. If a stranger was looking at me on the Tube, it was more likely that they were judging my clothes or the brand of phone I was holding. It felt a far cry from the openly racist signs that I'd heard pervaded London's pubs and cafés in the 1960s saying: 'No Blacks, no dogs, no Irish' (two out of three ticks against me!). At the same time, though, if I walked past a younger Black guy or an older man, we'd often find ourselves nodding to each other in a silent acknowledgement.

So, has my experience of growing up 'different' shaped who I am today? I suppose it played a part, but I think I emerged from the womb an irritatingly happy-go-lucky type. When it comes to exercise, I've found there are two types of confidence: firstly, having the confidence to make that initial step; and secondly, the confidence that comes *from* exercising – making gains in the right direction, however small. Hearing compliments, noticing changes within yourself, like feeling less sluggish and getting out of bed being less horrendous, and developing physical strength, are motivating. A growth mindset builds on small successes, adding to your confidence along the way.

> 'Sport has made me better in all facets of my life. It's taught me how to work hard to reach my goals. It's taught me how to handle disappointment and to be resilient. It's given me confidence and so many other skills that I can use throughout my life.'
>
> NIKKI CAUGHEY, FLY-HALF FOR IRELAND'S WOMEN'S RUGBY TEAM

Thinking with a growth mindset encourages resilience, and that will lead to success, whether that's at work, in our relationships or in our training. It's why, when I'm working with clients, I praise their efforts and determination as much as the results. And it's why I'll be giving you a bollocking if you fail to even try. We all need to take responsibility for our actions, so no more excuses: you *can* do it, you *will* do it. Here are a few quick places to start to help build up that emotional toolkit:

Resilience: A positive outlook on life is the secret to resilience. Being a moaning Michael will not just mean your nearest and dearest want to leg it every time they see you, but it can keep you stuck in negativity and thinking the worst is going to happen. Boost your resilience by changing your pattern of thinking. Basically, every time you start being down on yourself, reframe it. For example, if you feel you've made a mistake, remind yourself that you can learn from it and do something different next time. You'll need to do this deliberately at first, but the more you do it, the quicker it'll become second nature.

Surround yourself with good people: They will cheerlead you but also tell you when you're being an idiot! When I was playing semi-pro football, I had an agent who was full of shit. He never returned my calls as he had other, bigger-time players on his books, so I was left to flounder. Watch out for people like this in your life – they can crop up in many guises and ruin your confidence. Instead, find your tribe. Quality is much more important than quantity here. A handful of friends who you really care about and who care about you is far superior to a coachload of hangers-on.

> 'Embrace anyone who is willing to help you; always keep the door open.'
>
> GEMMA DAVISON, ENGLAND AND TOTTENHAM HOTSPUR FOOTBALLER

Ditch comparison: There will always be people who are stronger, fitter, richer and cleverer than you. True Fact. You may even be friends with some of them and find it envy-inducing to be around them, they're just so damn happy. But here's the thing: let them at it. Let them have their bigger house, their hotter husband or wife and their high-powered job. You don't have to keep up with them; they're doing their thing, you're doing yours. Free yourself from comparison. Channel your inner Elsa and let it go. I have definitely been guilty in the past of comparing myself with other weight-lifters and showing off online about how much I could lift. Often I would go beyond what my body was even ready to do, just to film my lifts in the hope of basking in validation from the virtual world. It took me a while to wise up, but now I'm all about doing what makes me happy. Follow your own path at your own pace.

Focus: Remember what you want to achieve and ignore any negative distractions so that you quieten your busy thoughts.

> 'It can be tough when your mind races in big moments. For me, it's about trying not to overthink situations, to focus on my process and the task in front of me. What helps me do this is to focus on my breathing, which allows me to stay present.'
>
> JOHNNY SEXTON, RUGBY CAPTAIN OF IRELAND AND WORLD RUGBY PLAYER OF THE YEAR 2018

Self-belief: After training so many clients, I've found that the transformation inside often begins with a physical change. Once you start feeling physically better and seeing your hard work pay off, it sparks change in other areas of life.

In her book *The Mind Monster Solution*, former boxer turned therapist Hazel Gale talks about how her negative inner critic would appear at crucial moments, like when she entered the boxing ring for a championship match, telling her she was going to fail. The pressure meant that she'd overthink all her signature movements and punches, which had previously been automatic. Have you ever heard that voice that says to you, 'What's the point going to the gym? You're never going to be able to be as fit as X', or the one tells you, 'Blow all those hard-earned savings on something you don't need', or 'Scroll mindlessly through your phone when you have a big work deadline'. These are the inner, niggling voices that represent our conscious or unconscious fear of failure, the "imposter syndrome" that stops you even trying. They can be your own worst enemy, almost willing you to fail. They are your deepest anxieties coming to the surface to scupper your best intentions, and they can creep up on you when you least expect it. I've seen it many times, where clients are making amazing progress, then *bam*, suddenly they're not showing up for training sessions. Or, at a higher level, it would be the equivalent of an athlete losing their nerve just before a big tournament and underperforming. I wish I could tell these destructive thoughts to go fuck themselves, but it's not always that simple. Instead, you might find it useful just to acknowledge them and remind yourself that, as Owen O'Kane says in his book *Ten Times Happier*, just because you think them, it doesn't mean they're true. Worrying about a problem doesn't make it go away; dwelling on it will only lead you to fixate, and that's a hard spiral to get out of. That's why thinking positively can have an incredible impact on our fitness success.

Remember that almost anything is possible, and that we're all on a journey where there'll be good and bad days. Is this all sounding very happy clappy? Do you want to punch me in the face? If so, just skip the rest of this section and jump straight to Part 2. If you're still with me, read on . . .

The power of language

How we talk to ourselves has a massive impact on our potential for success at the gym (and in everything we do). Using assertive language can make a huge difference. So, instead of saying, 'I'm going to try to go to the gym at some point this week,' say, 'I will be at the gym Tuesday, Friday and Sunday.' Rather than saying, 'I wish I could get in shape, but I've just got too much going on,' say, 'I am making changes to ensure I prioritise my health.' I know it sounds a bit 'out there', but the buck stops with you; failure's not an option.

Get beyond the stage of 'wanting' to do something. We often get stuck here, as if wanting is just a pie-in-the-sky dream that can't actually happen for real. 'I *want* a career change,' 'I *want* to find love,' 'I *want* to get fit' . . . It's not the rehearsal, people – make it happen.

And mind how you talk to yourself generally, especially if in the past you've been inclined to give yourself a knuckle-rapping. If you're someone who tells yourself, 'Oh, the gym's not for me' or 'I never did sport at school, I've never been good at it,' nip that in the bud right this minute, young lady/man. What you have or haven't done in the past can go fuck itself. This is about *now.* Exercise isn't for a 'type' of person – it's for absolutely everyone. Just because you were a champion at forging notes from your mum to get out of PE doesn't mean you won't absolutely nail a circus-skills class or enjoy hiking with friends. Don't limit your potential by telling yourself it's silly even to try. If you look after your body, it will extend to every part of life. If you respect yourself, others will do the same and that will feed your work, your relationships and your overall happiness.

ALL STATIONS TO MOTIVATION

> 'What you think, you become.
> What you feel, you attract.
> What you imagine, you create.'
>
> BUDDHA

Do what you love, love what you do

Back to this old chestnut! It may be a cliché, but it's still true that if you spend a large part of your time every day being exposed to things you don't like – your job, your home, your relationships, whatever – it creeps into your soul and any motivation you had dies a slow, painful death. Okay, obviously some things – that delightful prostate check or smear test – are unavoidable, but I mean your daily grind. If you're living for the weekends or feel like sobbing on a Sunday evening at the thought of work, that is not okay. Set the bar higher. You owe it to yourself to do something of value every day.

I have always thrown myself into work. As a teenager, I had various part-time jobs, like working in a department store alongside earning a few quid playing football. I never really wanted to grow up and get a 'real' job, and I've managed to do fairly well at avoiding anything that feels like 'work'. I've done a variety of things over the past few years to keep the wolves from the door, including making videos of pigeons shitting on stuff (I can't say that was a huge money-spinner, but I did have a laugh and it kick-started my presence on Instagram, which has opened so many doors for me). Something I've noticed with clients I've trained is that when they like what they do for a living, they're almost always more motivated to exercise, as if the contentment from one area of their life transfers to another. If you're feeling ground down by work, or anything really, it's harder to get your shit together with fitness. Once you do make that step, though, you won't know yourself for the positive changes that roll your way.

Something I've found is that, with work, as with life in general, keeping an open mind and adapting to curveballs is the way to go. Some people get fixated on linking achievement to age, i.e. 'By the time I'm 30, I must be at X level or have got Y promotion, otherwise I'll see myself as a failure.' The age/milestone mindset is a total fallacy; ditch it now and enjoy a feeling of weight being lifted off your shoulders. The danger of it is that you end up comparing yourself to friends (or more likely frenemies) and what they've 'achieved' rather than focusing on yourself. Secondly, it makes you obsess about the 'destination' rather than the 'journey'. Wealth and status are far from the only markers of success. Is reaching a certain level by the time you're 32 worth it if it means that for the five years preceding it, you're a slave to your job, stressed, overworked and with little time for friends and family? Shouldn't our timeline focus more on gaining experience, knowledge and skills rather than just a label or ranking? As the saying goes, you either have time or money. I'm not going to lie, both would be nice, but I reckon, where possible, choosing time is the way to go. Don't think this is a licence to sit on the sofa all day playing Minecraft; it's about striking a work–life balance.

While my career as a footballer (and then in rugby) didn't pan out quite the way I had imagined, I had to think of a Plan B – time to roll with the punches. My eldest daughter (aka Caramel Zeus) was born around this time and I had to keep her in the finest leather booties, to which she'd grown accustomed. I knew I wanted a career in fitness (plus I was far too unkempt for an office job – who'd have me?!) and, as I mentioned earlier, I had done my PT training and was hooked.

As tends to be the case in life, when one door closes,

another opens. Around this time, I started doing a bit of sports modelling, and one of my first big gigs was with Nike, standing in as a body double for Mario Balotelli. They were shooting a video for a trainers advert and, as luck would have it, we were the exact-same height and weight. Body doubling is a weird and wonderful profession (if you can call messing about on set a profession – and you probably can't). But having me double up for Mario meant that the production team could test all the shots, prepare the lighting and sort all the other behind-the-scenes stuff necessary for an ad to be filmed. This often takes a couple of days, but the star is only able to come for a couple of hours.

This led to some other big jobs with Mario and with some other incredible athletes, like Yaya Touré, Anthony Joshua and Usain Bolt. When they were appearing in campaigns, muggins here often came along for the ride. It was an incredible opportunity and always a laugh. I eventually had to stop because I was banging the gym so much that I was actually getting too big to stand in for some of them! I was getting bigger and bigger – great for me and my goals, but not so great for 'being' Mario or Usain. In some of the ad-campaign videos, it was the stars' heads cut out and pasted onto my body (as it was me who was on set for longer, practising the choreography), so video editors were having to make my arms smaller in post-production just so we matched.

I think it might have been a sign to wind it down. Doing the body-double gigs was awesome while it lasted, but there came a time when I thought it might be good to move on. I'm too old to be standing round a set all day as an extra – that's a young man's game! Time for the next chapter in my *Memoirs of a Meathead*. So, while it's important to feel you have direction in life, working towards goals, different things will work for you at different stages and your priorities will change. Having a flexible mindset will help you adapt to life's curveballs.

Haters are not motivators

Well, actually, I sometimes find they really are. When I get abuse online, it can spur me on, if only because I want to piss off the haters! For sanity, though, I reckon it's better to embrace the things you love and ditch what you don't. I have no time for people who can't have a laugh at themselves. Move away from these drains – they are motivational evil! – and find some radiators who are good craic (Irish for good fun). These are the people who you're pleased to see a WhatsApp from when their name flicks up on your phone, instead of wanting to ignore it. They're the ones you can be yourself with; they know you chat shit but don't care. The drains zap your energy; they only seem to talk about themselves and the drama that follows them around. The idea of a pint with them feels like an obligation to tick off your to-do list. Follow your instinct here and have a good old cull, Marie Kondo – style (except rather than asking if an old jumper sparks joy, you apply it your acquaintances). Goodbye, drains. Go and live in a bin, far away from me.

> 'Never give someone who is only temporary in your life's journey permanent status. Just because they say you can't, doesn't mean you won't.'
>
> ADEBAYO 'THE BEAST' AKINFENWA,
> STRIKER FOR WYCOMBE WANDERERS

Reframe your approach to working out

I hear a lot of excuses for not getting to the gym, and it's often from those who've started out going great guns, but after a few weeks their motivation is waning. They can't find the time. They've had a long day at work. There's a tonne of stuff they need to do at home. I'm not saying you don't need to listen to your body, of course you do. But cut the bollocks and ask yourself honestly: is avoiding exercise really doing you a favour? One way to help make time for fitness is to adjust how you think about it. Try not to see it as a chore but as a gift to your body and mind. It's not a punishment; you're working out not because you dislike your body but because you *respect* it. Look ahead at your week's schedule and slot in some gym time. Some weeks, when you're genuinely over-stretched, that might be a couple of 30-minute sessions; other weeks, you'll be able to make more time. This is about creating life-long habits so that exercise becomes a consistent part of your routine. When you find an exercise you love, this becomes so much easier.

> 'To have something you truly want, you have to be willing to do more than anyone else.'
>
> ANTHONY WATSON, ENGLAND AND BATH RUGBY PLAYER

'But, Black Zeus, I've never found an exercise I'm any good at! I'm shite at everything!' some of you might yelp. Chill your boots, because I am a Belieber that hard work counts for more than ability. Former table-tennis Olympian and sports writer Matthew Syed uncovered research in his book *Bounce* that supports practice and dedication, along with opportunity, outweighing natural talent. The cricket stars filing out at Lords or Paralympians playing wheelchair basketball are certainly talented, but what's often overlooked are the thousands of hours of practice they've put in to get them there. (Maybe not the cricket players, unless eating cream teas counts as practice. Is cricket even a sport?) Johanna Konta also had a first day, a first time she held a tennis racket, and no doubt she sank most of the balls into the net. These elite athletes haven't just fallen out of bed or inherited super-charged genes; they've made huge sacrifices, often putting their personal lives on the backburner to put in the hours. So, the more time you give to the exercise of your choice, the better you'll become. No one will do the work for you – there are no shortcuts – but it's much less of a grind when you find something fun. You *can* do it. So let this be a motivator and have faith that you can achieve fitness.

Make fit happen

If you've found all this theory I've been chewing your ear off about all well and good, but you want some practical motivation to get your ass out of bed each morning, here you go:

1. **Make time.** Why is it that we can make time to glance at our phones 6 million times a day, stay too late at work after an already long day or do a Netflix box-set binge most evenings? Why are we distracting ourselves with this crap rather than prioritising ourselves? Is looking at yet another Donald Trump meme

going to contribute to your health and happiness? Well, actually it might – that tangerine face is pretty funny. So, okay, you're allowed to watch one meme, but then get moving, pal. Time is our most precious asset, so protect it.

2. **Prioritise self-care.** You have a to-do list as long as your arm, your flat's looking like a crack den and the kids are hungry and feral. There's rarely a perfect time for exercise. So don't overthink it – just do it. Stressing about all your life admin will push exercise down the priority list, when it should be way up on top.
3. **Up and at 'em.** Play to your strengths and figure out when you're most likely to fit in a workout. Are you a lark or night owl? Many people find that as the day goes on and chaos reigns, it's harder and harder to get that workout ticked off the to-do list. If this sounds familiar, do yourself a favour and get into your workout gear as soon as you get up. You'll be more likely to get to it then. And if it's something you don't enjoy (although my mission is to help you find something you love or grow to love), getting it over and done with first thing – or 'eating that frog', as self-development guru Brian Tracy would say – will give you a spring in your step for the whole day.
4. **Having a focus** for whatever workout you're doing is essential. Rather than just rocking up and trying to wing it, it'll give you purpose. Get in, get out, you're done, *boom*. In Part 3, I give you workout ideas to follow, which will take the thinking out of it, if that's not your bag.
5. **Harness your hormones.** Exercise naturally releases

some banging hormones, such as dopamine and endorphins – your body's natural motivators – that will help do the job (see page 69 for more).

6. **Remember the good you're doing yourself.** If at first you see exercise as a punishment, just knowing that you're improving your strength, speed or endurance with every single movement you do is a powerful motivator.
7. **Don't let setbacks set you, er . . . back.** There'll be times you just can't prioritise your fitness and you'll get side-tracked due to some biggies in life like illness or injury, new parenthood, intense periods at work or general burnout. If possible, always try to keep your foot in the door by doing some form of exercise, even if it's much reduced. As with most areas of life, it's easier to pick something up again when you haven't totally left it behind. One way to do this is to adapt the intensity or frequency of your training to do the bare minimum. So, for example, if you're a middle-distance runner, you might try to squeeze in one or two 5k runs a week; if you can't get to football training for a few weeks, you could still do some light leg exercises at home (see page 149). The benefits might be more psychological than physical, and that's a good thing. However, if even this hasn't been manageable, don't berate yourself (what's the point?), just try to look after the things you *can* control (such as your diet and your sleep) until you can get back out there. When you have the time to focus once again, it's always possible to get back on track and it will be easier than you think, because the body remembers.

•

The life-changing power of routine

You've probably heard all the old clichés about getting started being the hardest thing or the first step on the road to success. While 'routine' sounds pretty boring, I do think that ingraining exercise into your day-to-day can be powerful, and it's surprising how quickly you can adapt to a routine. Basically, the more you make an effort to do something, like exercise, the quicker it becomes your 'normal' – great news for anyone wanting to get fitter and healthier.

Charles Duhigg, author of *The Power of Habit*, says that we are hardwired to form routines, that it's this that has allowed for the survival of the species – any mammals lacking good habits would naturally have died out. The part of our brain called the basal ganglia is our in-built mechanism for forming habits. It allows us to learn from past #fails and create smooth habits, even unconscious ones like putting one foot in front of the other. It's long been documented that very successful, productive people (like world leaders, top CEOs and winning athletes) rely heavily on ingraining habit in their day-to-day. Like my old mucker Barack famously wearing the same clothes every day (let's hope they were washed in between); he's assigning mundane tasks to habit so that he doesn't waste any energy thinking about trivial stuff. Others might eat exactly the same meals every day at the same times or wake up and go to sleep at the same time so as not to tire the brain out by giving it a choice. Being highly controlled in this way doesn't appeal to me, but I can see why it really works for many people. When we see exercise as a choice, it means there can be two options: do it or don't do it. So, if you eliminate choice and make it part of your habit, where you don't even question whether you're going to make netball practice tonight, you just do it.

Routines can make us more productive and disciplined. The more disciplined you are in one area of your life, the more ingrained it'll become. That doesn't mean you need to be a sergeant major about everything to do with exercise; it'll just make it easier to motivate yourself the more disciplined you become.

Carrying out simple daily tasks can make you more disciplined overall and therefore more likely to succeed. US Navy SEAL Admiral William H. McRaven (check out his YouTube speech to a graduating class at the University of Texas) says that creating daily habits can keep you on the straight and narrow, so that you get other shit done. Something like making your bed each morning can have a knock-on effect, spurring you on to tick off other things on the to-do list. I'm all for this approach if it gets you to the gym. Again, what works for one won't do the same for someone else. There's a bit of an obsession right now with being productive 100% of the time and it can lead to burnout. Do I make my bed every morning, with hospital corners? Fuck no. But I'm a freak who never needs any inspiration to smash the gym. My little routines include religiously making a protein shake as soon as I'm up in the morning as well as doing mobility stretches. And obviously I brush my teeth now and again.

If you've been a lazy sloth until now, waiting for a layer of fur to grow on your cup of tea from four days ago before bringing it to the sink (where you leave it languishing another week before washing it up), then check yourself. You might find that being a bit more #boom! with the basics will lead you to being more motivated elsewhere.

How to fit exercise into your daily life

I hear this constantly: you've no time! You're just so busy, poor love. Save it. Unless you're out rescuing orphans 24/7, I refuse to accept you can't work some fitness into your life. Depending on the type of exercise or training you do, even if it is on the more intense end of the scale, it'll likely still be a small proportion of your week. For example, an hour a day, four days a week is 2.4% of your waking time per week (God, that bit of maths took it out of me). That should be manageable for most people, especially as it's all about making choices to support your wellbeing.

This is where saying no to saying yes comes in. Psychologist Tony Crabbe explains why we should be less busy (basically, it's soul-destroying), and one thing he encourages us to think about is, if we say yes to something, it will mean saying no to something else. So, if I say yes to that drink with Kevin who-I-don't-even-like-because-he's-a-bore from the marketing department, it means saying no to getting to spin class or making the five-a-side football match after work. We know that life is a balancing act, we can't do it all and trying to do so just leads to brain fog. So, thinking in this way can help you assess what's important to you – what your priorities are right now. Busyness is an excuse, and living in a cloud of busy-bragging may make us think we're important and needed but it actually takes away control from us. Sometimes we have to say no to say yes. And by the way, I apply this also to anyone overdoing it on the exercise front – those who need to listen to their body and say no to a workout if they're feeling completely wrecked, and instead say yes to relaxing (by which I mean having an early night rather than hitting da club).

Your daily actions impact your life-long health, no doubt about it. And it doesn't have to be hours a day; it can be minutes. Below are some simple ways to move more. This isn't exactly Rocky Balboa running up those steps, just some easy swaps to make in your day-to-day which will complement any training. It's not rocket science, but taking every opportunity to move means it all adds up.

- If commuting by train or bus, stand up for the journey and get out a stop early to walk the rest of the way.
- Create a new playlist or download some new podcasts – having something different playing in your ears might help you move your arse more.
- Always take the stairs instead of the lift.
- Walk, and do so briskly! Before hopping into your car, ask yourself if you could realistically walk there – taking your kids to school on foot or walking to the shops are often just as convenient as driving; it's just a question of forming the habit.
- Sit down as little as you can: if working at a computer, try using a standing desk for part or all of the day; if you're meeting friends for a drink, stand by the bar, rather than pulling up a stool; if you're on the phone, take the call while walking, if possible.
- Do some simple stretching at home while watching TV.
- If you have kids, get outside and play with them as much as possible; you'll have fun and set a good example to them. When I'm doing daddy day-care,

a park trip with a football is almost always on the cards (for my sanity as much as keeping the kids occupied).

Let go of routines that aren't working

Just as you'll hopefully try to set up some new routines that will really support your health goals, saying 'so long, *adios*, farewell, *adieu*, *slán*' to some that aren't doing a whole lot for you should also be the case. I'm not talking here about reining in some vices like smoking or drinking wine by the pint (pack them in, for Gawd's sake), but you might have established some routines you think are keeping you on the straight and narrow but are actually just doing a whole lot of meh.

Gyms are full of old souls treading water, doing semi-effective workouts. Often they're people who've been going to the gym for years, and fair play to them for sticking at it, turning up two to three times a week, stuck in a routine that isn't pushing them forward, essentially meaning they're wasting their time. I've often spotted these poor chumps meandering from the cross trainer to the treadmill, and I think to myself, *They could spend half the time at each gym session but make it count far more.*

Often this is the most challenging group to motivate, and part of the reason for that is that they often cling to old advice that clearly isn't serving them that well any longer. This could be down to a type of cognitive bias, whereby you cling to the first piece of information you hear, seeing that as the king of the facts, which means you dismiss any other advice you receive afterwards. Let's say three years ago you had a one-to-one session with a PT during your gym induction. In this session, she suggested you focus on cardio training, such as running, to help achieve overall fitness and some weight loss. Your brain might have processed that as 'running is the best and only way I can lose weight and stay fit', and you might unknowingly cling to that 'truth' for the rest of time. Even when you see others at the gym attend a class or trying out new equipment, you remain resolutely committed to staying stuck in old habits. It's no one's fault, but without mixing it up a bit or setting yourself challenges, it's going to get pretty boring, and you'll be more likely to stop altogether.

So consider whether there are any vanilla routines you've outgrown and swap them for something more mint-choc-fudge-brownie. With sprinkles. And keep these tips in mind if you're struggling to try something new:

- **Say thanks to your old routine.** No, I haven't been sniffing too many gym fumes. Acknowledge that you've had some good times together but it's time to move on. It will help keep you in a positive mindset, ready to move forward towards new goals, without any recrimination of previous habits.
- **Little by little.** Change can be a drag, especially if you're someone who finds comfort in the safety net of a routine. If you have previously gone to the gym three times a week to use the treadmill, swap one of those sessions for a class and see how you feel. Little swaps can then be built upon.
- **Get a buddy involved.** I'll bet you have a friend, neighbour or family member who wants to get fitter, so join forces and try something new together. You'll find it less intimidating and more motivating if you have a Robin to your Batman or a Thelma to your Louise.

- **Think outside the box.** Dancing in a nightclub, wild swimming or trampolining with your kids are all brilliant ways to boost fitness. Eschewing typical exercise for something more offbeat can really help reinvigorate your routine.

GO SMASH YOUR GOALS

'A goal without a plan is just a wish.'

ANTOINE DE SAINT-EXUPERY

It doesn't matter what your current ability or experience is, you absolutely need a goal. It'll bring focus so that you achieve your aspirations. So, before you get that Lycra on, work out what you want to achieve. It may be that you want to get fitter, improve muscle tone, lower your blood pressure, have more energy or generally get stronger. Whatever your aim, having a specific goal (or goals) in mind will help keep your eyes on the prize. When I'm training clients, goal orientation is central. People often come to me with an aesthetic aspiration, saying they want to lose weight in order to look a certain way, or they might show me a pic of someone's body shape they admire. I don't think that's the healthiest way to approach a goal, so I always try to work with the client to readjust the goal towards something like getting stronger, being more being flexible and having more energy (and a by-product of this will be shaping up anyway).

I always have goals in mind when I'm training, both short-term and longer-term ones. I get closer to realising them by following a fairly rigid gym programme, but sometimes even the best intentions take time. Currently I'm playing the long game with my goal to deadlift 400kg. It may take a few years to get there, but it's still a massive focus point. With this being my overarching goal, I then focus on weekly and monthly smaller goals that all add up. This is a fairly detailed approached based on following an elite model of training, so don't worry – goal-setting can also be much simpler. I could probably achieve my deadlift goal sooner if I stopped reppin' pints and devoted all my time to training, but I want to have a life too. Everyone has a balance to strike.

How to set goals

Working out what you actually want to achieve can take a bit of thought. Try to visualise your goals. If you could wave a magic wand right now and transform yourself into your fitness avatar, what would be different? Could you run a half-marathon? Would you have joined a local basketball team, for the active element, but also for the banter? Or do you want to try something new, like being able to do a handstand after some time doing plyometrics? (BTW – that last one is a great show-off trick when you're pissed at a party . . .) Imagine your future self, having achieved new strength and confidence, and let this image give you a kick up the arse whenever you need it. The more you surround yourself with positive thoughts about your fitness success, the more likely you'll be to achieve. Play the long game, because the buzz you get from instant gratification doesn't last long.

I recommend setting three to five goals, with most of them focused on shorter-term ambitions and one or two on long-term ones. Challenge yourself by not listing any goals relating to how you look. As I've said before, things like weight loss aren't always an accurate measure of progress, particularly when you're building muscle, which is more dense than fat. It can be very demotivating for someone to work like a Trojan on their fitness regime, only for the scales to flash a number not inkeeping with their expectations. A set of scales can't tell you how you're feeling. On the flip side of that, I have worked with people who imagine that once they get the body of their dreams, they'll suddenly become happy and content. It doesn't work like that, I'm afraid. Often, when they do achieve their ideal aesthetic but their mental health and outlook remains the same, they're left deflated. This is the problem: if your self-worth is tied up with how you look, the aesthetic goalposts can frequently move and you might feel like you'll never get to where you want to be. But when your confidence comes from how you feel, it's a much healthier, more realistic way to live. In my experience of training people who are highly motivated by body image, changes are often not long-lasting.

Simple steps to setting smart goals

1. **Start small** – you can't eat an elephant in one sitting. You'll be much more likely to stick to goals that are realistic. If the idea of an hour-long swim or running a 10k is intimidating, begin by doing five minutes and don't think much further than that. There have been studies that show even 5–7 minutes of exercise a day is beneficial. Extreme lifestyle or dietary overhauls are rarely sustainable, so start gradually and work your way up.

2. **Set your goal for something very slightly out of reach** – nothing unimaginable, just something you can *quite* do at the moment. So, if you can currently do five press-ups, aim for eight, and keep readjusting as you progress. Set yourself challenges. They don't necessarily have to be big things like doing a triathlon – they could be holding a plank or a squat for five seconds longer each time. Your goals should evolve as your training progresses to avoid reaching a plateau.
3. **Keep your goals performance-based** and not about looking a certain way.

How to make your goals happen

- Make sure your training is specific to your goals (see my workout plans in Part 3 for more info). There's no point smashing weights at the gym if it's cardio strength you want to build.
- Do a little bit of research, prep so that you have a rough idea of what to expect of the training of your choice and whether it'll fit with your lifestyle. It will make it less daunting, if you're just getting started, if you have some idea of what it entails
- Write out your goals and stick the piece of paper somewhere in your home that catches your eye often (e.g. on the fridge or your bedside table). Let it serve as a daily reminder of why you're working so hard. Alternatively, you could keep a note of them on your phone.
- Share your goals with someone supportive and ask them to check in with you every week to see how you're getting on. Putting your goals out there will make you

more accountable, disciplined and likely to succeed. This is part of the reason you see me prancing about on social media shaking my glutes in spandex hot pants ... I need the accountability! (Or maybe it's not the accountability and I just like wearing spandex?)
- Think with a growth mindset – believe it will happen and it will. For me, knowing that I am stronger now than I was last week is a massive motivator that helps keep me committed to my goals.

How to measure progress

- Monitoring your progress isn't just essential for pushing yourself to the next level physically, it's also really motivating. Make a note of your workouts. For example, if you're at the gym, write down which weights or machines were used as well as duration times. Then you'll be able to see in black and white how you've progressed. Looking back on these notes will give you a boost if you need one.
- After every bit of exercise you do, have a brief think about how it went, whether you pushed yourself as hard as you could or, if you deliberately held back, think about how you might approach it differently next time. Check in to see how you're feeling both physically and mentally. The endorphins should be kicking in and you should finish feeling better than when you started (maybe not physically if you've destroyed yourself, but mentally at least!).
- Write down a list of milestones you want to achieve over the coming next month, three months and six

months. Revisit these regularly and celebrate every small win.

- The most important measure of progress is how you feel in yourself!

Advanced-level fitness

And what about those of you who are already very fit but want to take it to the next level, to reach peak performance?

Set yourself more ambitious goals: I realise this contradicts what I say to those starting out with new fitness plans, but as I strive for peak performance I sometimes set myself crazy goals. These goals might be several years in the making and seem ridiculously far away from my current ability, but I like having the bigger picture in mind and to envision the very highest ambitions for myself.

Total focus: If you really want to push your personal boundaries, you will have to prioritise and make sacrifices. Know that the pressure you put on yourself might increase, but at an appropriate level this can be a great motivator.

Look at your lifestyle: Make sure you are getting the nutrition and sleep you need, as well as coping with stress, otherwise you can spend all the time in the world exercising and you won't reach the top of your game.

Repetition: The more time, practice and effort you allocate to it, the more it'll pay off. Push yourself that bit harder in each session, perhaps staying a little longer than you ordinarily would. It's 'repetition' that elite athletes keep in mind.

Consistency: This is key, because it's hard to progress at a decent pace if your training schedule is erratic. Building a regular programme that is manageable, meaning you are able to train at a consistent pace each and every week, is far superior to exercising an extreme amount but less frequently.

No excuses

I'm going to get all international on your ass now, helping you to reignite focus if you've been ambling along in factory-setting mode. *Kaizen* is a Japanese principle used by the most successful global businesses, from Nike to Toyota, which is all about making continuous small improvements. The idea, a bit like marginal gains (see page 300), is that they all add up to a noticeable change. To apply this to fitness, first keep your goals in mind. For example, if you have a goal to exercise three times a week, then think about all the ways you can support yourself to make that happen. So, if you're working out early in the morning, you could have your kit laid out in your bedroom so that you jump straight into it when you wake up; you could have some breakfast or a smoothie already made up and waiting in the fridge; and you could have your bag for work packed and ready to go by the front door. Essentially, you're doing yourself a favour, making fitting in exercise as easy as possible.

Again, with *kaizen* in mind, you'd then try to anticipate any problems that might get in the way and nip them in the bud. It's a bit like doing a risk assessment of anything that might scupper your best intentions. Say you've booked an after-work gym class that starts at 6 p.m. You might check to ensure nothing will stop you leaving the office on time – oh, there's a 5 p.m. meeting; if that's likely to run on, can you bring your bag, coat etc. with you so you can leave for class straight from the meeting? Or, if you want to do an online yoga session at home but you don't want your kids interrupting, can you plan it for when they're less likely to bug you? Put everything in your diary or online calendar, as this will make it more concrete, like it's not an option. Basically – get your shit together, get organised, no excuses.

PART 2

YOUR BODY

Our bodies are amazing. They adapt to changes pretty quickly, which means it's never too late to start looking after them a bit better or pushing them towards a new challenge. It's almost mind-blowing when you start thinking about what's going on in your body when you exercise. I don't mean what you see on the surface – like looking in the mirror at the results of your hard work, when you start seeing all those hours pay off; I mean the incredible biological and chemical changes happening. My obsession levels have reached the point where I'm not that bothered about how I look – I rarely check my reflection in the mirror; my reason for lifting is how it makes me feel, and a big inspiration for me is thinking about the invisible stuff going on behind the scenes in my body.

For years, when I was playing football, I'd go to the gym without a real understanding of what my body was actually doing there. It was all about seeing the external results, like my arms and legs getting bigger. But knowing what's going on under the skin can help us get prepared for the physical demands of training – with this in mind, there'd be no point in me spending time at the gym doing cardio. In fact, that would damage my strength training. Changes occur to our body during exercise, and understanding these help us to optimise peak performance, especially during training, while making sure we exercise safely.

SPORTS PHYSIOLOGY 101

I'm always in awe of the body's natural ability to adapt. The way in which it works hard behind the scenes, in response to your exertions, is a beautiful thing – it's like it's willing you forward! I remember first covering different aspects of physiology when I was studying to become a PT; it was a real 'Aha' moment. It was the first time I'd felt gripped by learning. I was never that interested in school; I was always messing about, never taking schoolwork seriously. I just wasn't the studious type – textbooks, blackboards and homework bored me to tears. I was far too hyper for all that! I must have been a nightmare to teach. But the body – that's a subject I couldn't get enough of.

Our body's systems work together to facilitate exercise and adapt to it. Below are the highlights you need to know, and (weirdo that I am) I sometimes think about the amazing things these systems are doing, all of their own accord, while I'm training.

The musculoskeletal system

This is made up of two systems: the muscular and the skeletal (you didn't see that one coming, did you?). Essentially, it's what's holding us up, what supports us and controls our movements. Our bodies are composed of muscles, cartilage, tendons, nerves, ligaments, organs, joints and hard and soft connective tissue, formed within and around the skeleton, which is providing the support.

Physical activity is essential for bone health and for maintaining bone strength (so you really are being a 'lazy bones' when you don't get out to exercise). Parts of our skeleton even continue growing until we're around twenty-five years old. Our bones work pretty hard for us, keeping us stabilised, moving us around, acting as a shock absorber and protecting our vital organs, so when you exercise you're doing them a favour.

If you want to look after your musculoskeletal system, exercise is non-negotiable, and if you shy away from it now, you will feel it later on in life. It can help keep away joint stiffness, promote joint stability and mobility, build muscle strength, increase ligament and tendon strength, and increase blood supply to muscles through building the number and density of capillaries.

Muscles

It can sometimes be easy to overlook the importance of the purpose muscles are actually serving – in addition to being Exhibit A at your private gun show! This book is pretty muscle-focused – how to develop them, push them and help them recover – so let's have a look at what's going on in there.

There are over 600 muscles in our body, making up almost half our body weight. Muscles are composed of water, protein, fat and glycogen, which make up cells and combine to form thousands of tiny fibres. It's the nerves within the muscle fibres, specifically the proteins myosin and actin, which make the muscle contract, and how strong your muscle is depends on how many muscle fibres are present. The body metabolises food to create adenosine triphosphate (ATP), which carries the energy that fuels the muscle to move.

There are two types of muscle fibre: slow-twitch (type 1), which facilitates endurance-type activities like long-distance running, meaning it tires less quickly but doesn't pack a punch; and fast-twitch (type 2), which allows for shorter, more impactful exertions but can't be sustained over a long period. Slow-twitch fibres contain mitochondria, which convert oxygen and nutrients into ATP.

Motor units

These are made up of neurons and muscle fibres and, put simply, their job is to work together to make a muscle contract. These dudes are important to know about because they work by receiving signals from the brain, and the more active you are, the more muscle fibres will be stimulated. The higher the number of motor neurons activated, the stronger the muscle will be (this is called maximal motor unit recruitment). Motor units become dormant through inactivity (the phrase 'move it or lose it' is spot on), but the good news is that once you start exercising, these begin to fire up again. It's why those who start hitting the gym often see big results in the early weeks – it's like their motor units are waking up after a nap.

Hypertrophy

By progressively putting muscles under strain, for example when weightlifting, the cells and tissues within the muscles repair, then grow in size and become stronger. So, when people talk about building muscle, what they actually mean is increasing muscle fibre distribution and thickness by adding more myosin filaments (marginally less catchy than the term 'build muscle', I'll admit). Depending on the type of exercise you're doing (more on this in the next section), you will be targeting different muscle groups, and muscle growth can be supported through your diet.

The respiratory system

During exercise the brain sends signals to the respiratory system to increase breathing, inviting in more oxygen and getting rid of carbon dioxide. Over time, the benefits of exercise can lead to improved brain function and concentration. Here's how exercise impacts the respiratory system:

Lung capacity

Physical exertion puts pressure on the lungs and, over time, with regular exercise, the lungs will adapt, working hard to move more air in and out. This in turn affects your breathing rate; as you become more fit, oxygen-rich blood will be pumped around your body and you'll huff and puff less. You might have noticed, if you've ever reduced or stopped regular exercise, that even after just a few weeks you run out of puff much more quickly.

Respiratory muscles

The intercostal muscles and diaphragm get better at breathing air in and out as exercise increases blood flow. Cardio improves their endurance, whereas strength training grows their size and power, allowing expansion into the chest.

Alveoli and gas exchange

Tiny alveoli cluster throughout the lungs and are surrounded by capillaries, exchanging oxygen and carbon dioxide (a waste product) within the blood stream.

Capillarisation

When muscles are at work, like when they're exercising, they need more blood. Capillaries are blood vessels that help bring blood to and from the muscles, supplying them with oxygen and nutrients. Capillary density is the number of capillaries feeding a muscle, and this density increases with regular aerobic exercise in a process called capillarisation, in which the capillary network expands and grows even more blood vessels. In practical terms, this additional oxygen supply boosts energy and fights tiredness while decreasing pain and discomfort (by reducing delayed onset muscle soreness). The excess post-exercise oxygen consumption (EPOC) is the amount of oxygen needed by the body after working out to restore it to its regular state.

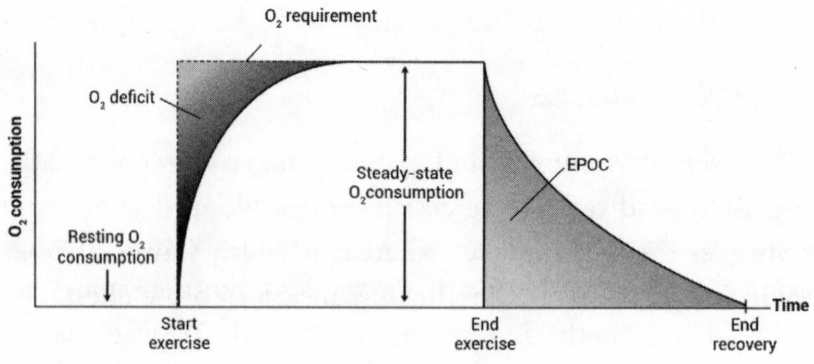

EPOC curve

The central nervous system (CNS)

The CNS is made up of the brain and spinal cord, and it controls most functions of the body. There's still a lot that's yet to be understood about it, but in simple terms, when you exercise your body, your CNS is exercising too. Exercises, particularly strength-training ones, send signals from the part of the body you're working to the brain, and vice versa. Amazingly, this means that, for people unable to do certain movements (such as those who are bed-bound), their cellular chemistry actually changes because their body hasn't been able to send signals to the brain. It's thought that the purpose of these signals is to build neural cells, essential for a healthy brain and nervous system. It's mad to think that until relatively recently the body and brain were being treated as separate entities.

When it comes to exercising, you need to work with the CNS, and a lack of awareness about it can be really detrimental. In fairness, it's an often-overlooked subject, so it may be that this is all news to you. Ideally you want the communication lines between your body and brain to be ship-shape. Additionally, your brain has to be on board with what your body is about to do – if it senses danger, it will reduce the strength available to you. For example, if you are doing a squat and the brain has an inkling your joint may not be strong enough to withstand that manoeuvre without injury, it will hold back on the amount of force it sends. Basically, your CNS has your back. Strength training, such as powerlifting, works the CNS by shocking it. When you follow a training programme that changes the stimulus frequently, it means the body responds by switching on motor units, getting you stronger more quickly.

CNS fatigue

This is when our ability to activate a muscle is impaired, and it's associated with chemical changes in the brain. It can be caused by over-training, not resting for long enough between workouts, or general stress and exhaustion. If you're suffering from CNS fatigue you may feel lacking in motivation or unable to fully activate certain muscle groups. You may notice a drop in your performance for no other obvious reason, and it may prolong your recovery time.

The cardiovascular system

Think of this as your body's Uber, transporting blood, oxygen, hormones, cells and nutrients around the body while removing waste. It's basically a Toyota Prius.

The heart

For some, it's a romantic date night with their partner – drinks and a candlelit dinner – but for me, what's worth getting worked up about is . . . the left ventricle. Those blood-red chambers, those teasing veins and arteries, the rhythmic beat – *ba-bum, ba-bum, ba-bum.*

Is this why I'm single? Possibly.

The left ventricle is the heart's main pumping chamber, and taking care of it by exercising can make this muscle get stronger – so it's not all about the biceps, people. Improvements can happen within a matter of weeks, meaning if you start exercising today, your heart might be likely to enjoy the benefits in a month or so.

During exercise there's an increase in cardiac stroke volume (the amount of blood pumped from the left ventricle with each beat) and heart rate, and over time, with continued exercise, this tends to reduce the resting heart rate (RHR). During cardio-based training, the heart beats faster, increasing the amount of blood pumped through the body. This increased circulation brings oxygenated blood to your muscles.

The heart adapts to exercise by becoming more efficient at circulating blood because it doesn't have to work so hard. Long-term benefits of keeping yourself in shape therefore include reduced risks of heart disease and lower blood pressure.

Hormones and neurotransmitters

These are chemicals produced by the endocrine system, glands that produce hormones and send messages to different parts of the body via the blood stream. They work in a complex way, impacting key functions of the body such as brain development, blood pressure, hunger, growth, reproduction and metabolism. When it comes to training, there are key hormones which are released by the body that serve to boost your workouts (another sign that your body wants you to move!). It's one of the reasons experts often recommend exercise as part of a wider care plan to those suffering from conditions like depression or anxiety. Here are just some of the hormones and neurotransmitters whose effects you might feel when you exercise, proving that the mental benefits of working out are every bit as real as the physical ones.

Harness these and you should naturally feel more motivated to work out:

- **Endorphins:** These are the body's natural mood lifters, which can also reduce the perception of pain. Some say that the effects of endorphins are similar to morphine. Yes, please.
- **Dopamine:** There's a reason this is known as the 'happy hormone' as it releases feelings of pleasure and motivation. A dopamine hit might help you get to the gym in the first place, while after your workout you'll be rewarded with endorphins.
- **Serotonin:** Another feel-good chemical that gives an overall sense of wellbeing. It's also key for sleep. Exercise is a brilliant way to produce serotonin and regulate it, and it also helps make melatonin (another hormone that promotes sleep).
- **Oxytocin:** This is the so-called 'love hormone'. It plays a much bigger role in women's bodies (where it helps support childbirth and breastfeeding) than men's, but it's also a hormone that is released during physical activity, particularly if you're enjoying the exercise. When stress levels are up, this hormone decreases.
- **Cortisol and adrenaline:** These are the body's stress hormones, activating the parasympathetic nervous system and the 'fight or flight' response. To a certain extent, the body interprets exercise as a form of stress. However, as you become fitter, exercise actually reduces the levels of cortisol and adrenaline.
- **Testosterone:** This sex hormone is released during exercise, particularly during weightlifting, and one of

its functions is that it helps build muscle. It's present in both men's and women's bodies (peaking around ovulation during the menstrual cycle in the latter). Interestingly, it's thought that testosterone levels naturally decrease when a man has kids.

Energy systems

You cannot underestimate the importance of energy-system training. Understanding what's going on behind the scenes when you work out will massively benefit the results you get, making your training much more efficient and effective. It will also impact your big-picture training programme, such as dietary needs and rest requirements. The truth is that I've seen people spending hours at the gym every week and not see much to show for it all because they're not working in tandem with their energy system. Is this all sounding very crystals, chakras and essential oils? Let me stop you right there, because there ain't nothing woo-woo about this.

There are three systems in the body that transfer energy around, enabling us not just to exercise but to live. These three systems all work together, often overlapping, and depending on the kind of activity you're doing, your body will use one system more than the others at any one time. Metabolic pathways cause chemical reactions in our bodies that produce ATP (adenosine triphosphate). ATP is a chemical produced in our cells that releases energy around the body, driving movements such as muscle contraction. Strenuous activity uses it up and it's then replaced by lactic acid. You can train and develop these systems to boost your workout, becoming as powerful as possible.

1. Anaerobic Alactic System (ATP-CP)

This system creates brief bursts of energy, allowing very intense and efficient movements. These stores are limited, so can't sustain intense muscular contraction, but through periods of rest can quickly build back up. The source of this energy is phosphocreatine (I'll be coming back to this, so stay awake) and it comes from within the body's tissue. The point of developing anaerobic (i.e. exercise that doesn't rely on oxygen to break down glucose) power is to strive for peak power for a very short burst of around 5–10 seconds. Think athletics such as the high jump or games like golf.

2. Anaerobic Lactic System (glycolytic pathway)

Like the ATP-CP system, this is responsible for immediate energy bursts, but this has a higher capacity for more sustained exercise, potentially lasting around 10 seconds to two minutes. It breaks down glucose in the body into lactic acid and fuels medium- to high-intensity training such as bodybuilders doing a 50m freestyle swim. The release of lactic acid then slows down the exercise, causing muscle pain, meaning it can't be sustained for too long. Picture a 400m runner – they burst out of the starting line into a sprint, full of beans, and their aim for the race is to try to keep to this pace as far as they can. Towards the end of the race, you'll see them getting out of breath, becoming visibly fatigued and looking more physically uncomfortable, which is the lactic acid building up in their muscles, slowing them down. They'll finish the race slower than when they started, but it's the runner who slows the least who'll win. After two or so minutes, the lactic system will give way to the aerobic system. It can regenerate ATP without the need for oxygen.

3. Aerobic System

This efficient system facilitates longer but lower-intensity outputs such as team sports like rowing, long-distance running or swimming (if you're doing gentle-paced laps). It requires high levels of oxygen and it can be sustained longer as a result – at least a couple of hours, though at a much lower power-level than your maximum. Oxygen flowing through the muscles drives recovery and so this system can work in tandem with the other two, as the aerobic system enables you to recharge your ATP-CP. So, while you might think that working your aerobic energy system is mainly a means to getting fit (in the cardio sense of the word), harnessing this system can also aid your muscle recovery when doing types of training that are anaerobic-based. It helps recharge and recover phosphates, which in turn helps build muscle, promotes bone health and generally supports wellness.

Some of the workouts I go into later on very much rely on one of these systems being predominant, such as shot put or javelin using the anaerobic alactic system, whereas others, like tennis, use two. Some exercises, like rock climbing and boxing, even use all three. Knowing which system is at play will focus your attention on whether your aim is to, for example, build strength, endurance or speed.

Regular exercise, particularly aerobic exercise, trains the body to increase blood flow to the muscles, improving their ability to draw on oxygen and become more efficient. Despite the impressive capability of muscles that have been exposed to lots of cardio training, they don't generally grow much in size or strength, which is why sports people like footballers are super-fit but not particularly muscly. And it's the reason I'm the opposite.

A couple of years ago, I took part in a hike up Everest in the vast great outdoors, surrounded by the most unbelievable scenery. I had lovely intentions of doing some cardio training to help prepare myself, which of course went out the window. I arrived at the Himalayas thinking *How hard can it be? I'll be grand.* So there we were, all ready to go, with all the gear, in my tip-top hiking boots, all set to fly up the 'hill' without breaking a sweat. As the hike went on, and with the altitude change, I died a death. I could barely keep up, all because I am so unused to that kind of exercise, which relies on much more efficient oxygenation of the muscles. The gas exchange – which brings oxygen from the lungs to the bloodstream and sends carbon dioxide back the other way – was so much less efficient for me. And the high elevation made everything worse – it's why many professional runners sometimes go to places of high altitude for training periods, to better their lung capacity and to build their endurance. There were grannies, better prepared aerobically and more used to the altitude, strutting past me while I'd be grasping at a rock, gasping for air.

It did bring it home and I made a plan to do more cardio, mainly by using a rowing machine – not so much that it would interfere with my power-lifting training, but enough to boost blood flow and improve endurance.

Have I bored you sh*tless with this biochemistry lesson? I know I've whittled on a bit but, I promise, having a basic understanding of your body will mean your workout will work a lot harder for you.

WOLF OR BEAR?

As I've said before, there isn't a one-size-fits-all when it comes to fitness and training; it all depends on what you want to achieve and what you enjoy doing. Similarly, people respond to exercise in different ways, based on various factors, including genetics. For example, I can deadlift 335kg, but my toddler could probably out-run me! Whereas when I played football and rugby, I could run 10k during a match without breaking much of a sweat, but I was way less strong.The shit's about to get real here: we're going to find an activity to suit you, and you'll have a ready-made plan and practical advice for your chosen workout. There may be crossover between choices, and these may change in the future. For example, right now, you might be looking to meet some more people, in which case joining a local team might be the way to go. Or maybe it's the opposite – you have a really hectic job where people are up in your bidness all day, so perhaps doing something mentally restorative like yoga will be the right tonic.

Cardio v strength

I can't believe we've got this far into the book without discussing the importance of embracing your spirit animal (a concept which is 100% scientific and evidence-based). This is what I call the Wolf or Bear test. Do you want to be fast, lean and light on your feet, agile like a wolf? Or do you want to be robust, muscular and forceful like a bear? Or somewhere in between, like a . . . badger? No, that's not quite right. Basically what I'm trying to say is, depending on the type of sport you do, your body will react in different ways. So, consider how you want to feel and what you would like to achieve through your workout regime (see Jump, Play, Stretch, Lift on page 87 for inspiration).

Cardio training is an umbrella term for a variety of activities that can vary in intensity and duration. During an aerobic workout, muscles increase their use of oxygen as they generate more energy to allow them to contract. The red blood cell content is increased, which in turn boosts blood volume. The beauty of cardio is that you'll build endurance through your training and you'll notice it in everyday life too – you'll feel more energised in daily tasks and you'll be nimble as a wolf.

Then there's strength training, also called resistance training. I could wax lyrical about this all day, as it's pretty much my life and how I spend most days. I love this type of training, particularly in the form of powerlifting. If I had to rate my love for lifting along with that for my kids . . . well, I honestly wouldn't like to explore where that would go. The thought of resistance training might conjure up images – if you're getting a flash-visual of meat-heads posing at bars, wearing white V-neck T-shirts three times too small for them – but it's not *all* about that either (though, in fairness, there's a bit of that going on). There's been an increased take-up among other groups in this type of training who are trying it out to boost overall health or complement other training they're doing. It's scalable, meaning it's not all about getting so big you can turn over a truck (although that's awesome, needless to say). Strength training can be just as effective at a much lower level. For me, it's all about the bear.

There are sports that combine the best of both – a bear-wolf if you will, a jack of all trades. If you've ever watched the Olympic cyclists going all out doing sprints in the velodrome, you'll see they have massive legs – that's because their training combines cardio and strength.

You could combine a session or two of strength training a week with a more cardio-based exercise, and that's great too. It probably means you won't be reaching elite levels in either, but you'll be an all-rounder, and there's a lot to be said for that.

Here are some of the many benefits of strength and cardio training:

Cardiovascular training

- Helps maintain healthy weight
- Strengthens the heart and lowers blood pressure
- Improves joint mobility, helping prevent injury
- Releases feel-good hormones
- Helps relieve stress and improve focus

Strength training

- Builds muscle mass
- Helps maintain bone density
- Increases range of motion and flexibility
- Reduces injury
- Burns calories both during and after a workout
- Reduces stress

FIND YOUR THING

Whether you want to build muscle, lose weight or generally have more energy, let's find a workout for you. Tuning into what you enjoy and what your body gravitates towards is popularly called 'intuitive fitness'. It makes sense if only because if you don't enjoy the exercise you're doing, you're unlikely to stick at it. If you're currently in a situation where you do a bit of exercise but dread it or feel apathetic while you're there, then DO SOMETHING ELSE, please. If your heart's not in it, your body won't be either.

During my football days, when I was playing for Grays Athletic in the fifth-tier Conference League (as it was known then), we had a pre-season friendly against Tottenham Hotspur at their training ground. At the time, they had some amazing strikers, like Adel Taarabt and Giovani dos Santos, and perhaps unsurprisingly they beat us 4–0. I was playing up front for Grays and dos Santos was my counterpart for Spurs. He was incredible – running rings around our defence, in one instance nutmegging our best defender, quickly flicking the ball back over his head and running on with the ball to score. I was in awe watching such skill, and it was a lightbulb moment because I suddenly realised I'd never be as good as that, no matter how hard I trained. Sometimes blind optimism and hard graft isn't enough. It was a turning point for me, as I realised I probably wouldn't get to that level and it was time to call it a day.

'We all have our own story to tell and mine of being a footballer has had its ups and downs, like any other person in this world. What I've learned along the way is invaluable to me. Always remember that a professional is just an amateur who hasn't quit.'

ADEBAYO 'THE BEAST' AKINFENWA,
STRIKER FOR WYCOMBE WANDERERS

Just to be clear – this isn't to say that if you're not amazing at a certain type of exercise you should sack it off. That's not at all what I mean, because if you're doing an activity that brings you happiness, of course it doesn't matter if your skills are less than perfect. I had lost my passion for playing football at that stage. If I was still loving putting my boots on every day, I would have been proud to play in any league, no doubt about it.

What are you looking for?

Strength	*	Powerlifting
Build muscle	*	Bodybuilding
Explosive power	*	Plyometric training
Increased stability	*	Calisthenics/gymnastics
Endurance	*	Running
Whole-body fitness	*	Boxing
Mental clarity	*	Yoga
Sociability	*	Football
Camaraderie	*	Rugby
Complete fitness	*	CrossFit

Have a think about the type of fitness or the psychological benefits you'd like to gain from exercise (there are some listed above) and this will help you focus on what to try. Depending on whether you're up for a challenge, you may want to choose something to push you out of your comfort zone (for example, trying a team sport if you've previously never done one). While I do like to advocate that variety is the spice of life, for some of you, doing any bit of exercise is already pushing you outside your comfort zone. If that's the case, then at the start you might be doing yourself a favour by choosing something vaguely familiar (or the least intimidating!), so perhaps start with jogging rather than base jumping for the time being.

Coming up in the next section are ten disciplines, each and every one with the potential to change your life for the better. These plans can be scaled up or down depending on your level of experience, getting you started if you're a beginner (or, in the case of some of the weightlifting plans, helping you progress to the next level). They're not exhaustive (each discipline would require its own book for that!), but they give you a flavour of how they'll get you fit.

NEWBIE AT THE GYM

A lot of the workouts that follow are gym-based, but I want you to forget any preconceptions you have around the gym. The days of it being just for posing bodybuilders are long gone, and you're as likely to see some happy retirees when you're there as you are anyone else. I've spent much of the past twenty years in the gym and feel pretty at home there – the noise of iron clanking is more soothing to me than birdsong!

When you're new, the gym can feel a little intimidating – everyone seems to know what they're doing and you might feel way out of your comfort zone. Now I don't want to scare you off, but think of your gym as you would ... the slammer. I needn't tell you what happens to white-collar-crime Johnny – he's arrived to the clink radiating fear. He nervously watches everyone pacing about during yard time, unsure of himself and his new home – and the other inmates can smell it a mile off. He's wondering who he can trust – the roaming wardens (the PTs)? The lifers (heavy-lifters)? Okay, I'm not saying you need to go all *Shawshank*, but if you're rocking up at a gym for the first time, confidence is key – but there's no need to run your water flask up and down the bars of the lockers like an inmate's tin cup. The law of the jungle applies here. If you are feeling apprehensive, like you're standing out like a sore thumb, not knowing what to do or how to use the equipment, it will affect your sense of purpose and, in turn, your performance. But don't worry, this isn't about a fake-it-till-you-make-it vibe; it's simply about having a plan.

Everyone has had a first day and, in reality, for the most part, people are focusing on themselves at the gym. Yes, there are a few peacocks parading their Lycra-clad plumage, Alphas sizing up the competition, trying to be the big dudes on campus. But that's on them. Recently, when I started going to my new gym, I had those inner flutterings of 'I'm new here, I'm not familiar with the machines, I'll have to get my head round how it all works ...' The first session is always the hardest, so once you've tackled that, you'll be out of the starting blocks.

Unleash the beast

Whether you're a seasoned gym-goer who's a ringer for Arnie circa *Pumping Iron* or a total rookie, we all need a plan to follow to keep us focused and prevent us gormlessly wandering round the gym floor. In the next section I give weightlifting newbies a plan for the first session, but before the actual workout there's some simple prep to do to get you started. Firstly, arrange an induction. This tends to be the protocol at most gyms, where one of the staff will give you a guided tour, showing you what's what. Even if you've been going to the gym for some time, ask for a refresher induction – you don't have to be a newbie to benefit from this. It's a great opportunity to get the lay of the land and watch demos of the machines. Don't be afraid to ask questions – you are learning the ropes and will do so quickly, even quicker if you are proactive. People want to help – they are *there* to help, as well as to keep you safe.

Knowing what you want to achieve will inform what you actually do at the gym. As a general starting point, though, if you are weightlifting you'll want to build up your strength, and resistance training is the first port of call. Workouts can initially focus on the whole body, and as you go along you can start mixing up these sessions, targeting specific areas of the body through a volume programme. As your plan evolves, you can go from machine to free weights, but starting gradually (don't worry, you'll still be challenged!) will prepare body and mind, laying solid foundations. And it means you won't be carted off to A&E when you keel over.

How to get started:

- Begin every workout with some warm-ups to prepare your body.
- Keep an open mind by trying out different aspects of the gym, such as classes (which are often included in membership fees). Mixing it up can be a good way to introduce you to different options.
- If you are weightlifting, start with machine weights, easing your way in and protecting your core. Going straight into free weights could cause injury. Remember your machine manners: if you're waiting for a machine to become free, just ask the user how many sets they have left and you can fill in your waiting time with some other exercises.
- Whether you're going to classes or staying on the gym floor, don't kill yourself on day one, but keep going. It will get easier and you'll grow in confidence once you've made that first step.
- At the start, aim for 45 minutes to an hour per session, three times a week, working your way up gradually.

Your Session 1 plan of attack

We should all be incorporating some resistance training into our exercise routine (see page 192 for the list of benefits). This plan is a great introduction and resistance-training all-rounder – a straightforward full-body workout for your first session. It should take around 45 minutes to an hour and you can do this on three days over your first week. Arrive at the gym with this plan and you'll have a sense of purpose straight away.

Here are three exercises for mobility to prepare you:

Hip opener

Frog stretch: Get onto all fours and slowly move both knees out to the sides. Ease into this stretch if it's new to you. Flex your ankles and push your feet out to the sides (it's the insides of your feet that should be against the floor). Again, move them out only to as far as they want to go (it will get further with time). Stretch your forearms out, placing them flat on the floor, palms down. Stay here for as long as is comfortable, and when you're ready to release, do so slowly.

Thoracic spine stretch

Prayer stretch: Come down on your knees in front of a bench or a chair (as if you were about to pray). Place your elbows on the bench, with your arms reaching up towards the ceiling, palms together. Your eyes should be looking down at the floor, keeping the spine and the neck aligned (rather than your neck and head bending towards the floor). Hang out here for as long as is comfortable. You can make this stretch even better by holding a broomstick or a PVC pipe between your hands, with your palms facing the ceiling in a bicep curl position.

Core exercise

Plank: Get into a press-up position with your palms on the floor under shoulder level and lower your elbows to the floor. Your legs should be stretched out and activated, with your toes pushing into the floor. Engage your core muscles and tense your glutes. Hold for as long as you can.

EXERCISE	***REPS***	***SETS***
Leg press machine	12	4
Chest press machine	12	4
Leg extension machine	12	4
Low rowing machine	12	1
Leg press machine	12	4

Remember, before you start using these machines, ask a PT at the gym to show you how they work and to watch you as you first go on, to ensure your position and movements are correct.

Black Zeus's dos and don'ts of the gym

DO

- Have a simple plan from the get-go. This can evolve as you make progress.
- Ask questions and know that there are people whose job it is to help you.

- Go at your own pace. Quicker doesn't necessarily mean better. Start sensibly and build up gradually.
- Watch and observe the experts such as the PTs.
- Remember that you have as much of a right to be at the gym as anyone.
- Stay positive – your body is amazing and you will soon see the results of all your efforts.
- Leave your ego at the door.

DON'T

- Imitate the crazy exercises you see others (er . . . like me) doing on social media. In time, you'll be able to build up to these, as your body gets stronger.
- Compare yourself to others at the gym – this is about YOU, not anyone else.
- Go straight to the free weights – stick to the machine weights to start with.

I'm a big believer in happiness coming from tackling things head-on. If you put the effort in, you *will* see results. And you may surprise yourself by finding you love it. I've seen so many supposed gym-haters converted.

PART 3

TIME TO TRAIN

Jump: CrossFit and HIIT, boxing, running, plyometrics
Play: football, rugby
Stretch: yoga, mobility, calisthenics, gymnastics
Lift: bodybuilding, powerlifting

Right, MoFos, we've come to the part where I'm going to whet your appetite, hopefully inspiring you to give one (or several) of these disciplines a go. There are of course thousands of types of exercises out there, some mainstream, others offbeat, but all with benefits. Don't feel you need to limit yourself to the ones I cover here; the idea is that you can test the water, glimpse the type of thing you might enjoy and take it from there depending on what you want to get from it. The ten disciplines in this section are ones I've tried myself and loved at various points of my life. Many will be familiar to you while others are a bit more unusual. Ones like football I was doing since I could walk, while others, like plyometrics, were introduced to me to help support my other training, like powerlifting. Similarly, I'm relatively new to yoga, so even though I can't claim to be an expert, I can vouch for it improving my range of motion, facilitating my work in the gym.

The options covered in this section firstly focus on aerobic training and then move into resistance training using body weight and free weights, though some, like CrossFit and boxing, incorporate both cardio and strength-training components. Many of the exercises at the start offer an alternative to the gym-based ones that follow later, and instead they get you out into the fresh air, into parks, country lanes or neighbourhood pitches, year-round. They generally don't require memberships or classes to book, are inexpensive and a brilliant way to let off steam. There are team sports in here too, as games like football and rugby (which, as you might have noticed already, are big passions of mine) are incredible routes to fitness. They sometimes these don't even feel like exercise because there are so many other aspects taking your focus, such as a sociable angle or community element.

I've written about the physical benefits of being active, how the body absolutely needs to move and be challenged several times a week. I've also talked about how exercise supports good mental health, making you more cheerful, resilient and confident. There's something else I want to mention, and that's loneliness.

Loneliness is an epidemic on the rise in our world of Insta, TikTok and YouTube – 9 million people in the UK say they're lonely, and the impact of that on their mental health must be massive. There's a real irony that as we become more glued to social media (yup, that's me!), the more followers we have, the lonelier we might become. It's a feeling of alienation and isolation that can really take its toll, grinding us down and making people become more insular, damaging self-esteem and general wellbeing. When I first moved to London, I had no friends; it was through playing football and later rugby, and joining a gym, that I met people. Sport was my lifeline. You can live in a busy city, have a big circle of friends, a tight-knit family and decent colleagues yet still be lonely, because it's all about the quality of the connections at any given time. And if we're feeling a bit low anyway, loneliness can really ramp up, increasing the risk of depression and anxiety. There are some great initiatives out there that aim to keep folks linked up – in Dublin they even have benches painted a certain colour that, when you sit on them, signal you're up for a chat with a stranger.

There are loads of good ways to combat loneliness. There are schemes that encourage meeting neighbours and sharing skills, and some socially distant ones came into their own during the COVID pandemic. It's a beautiful thing to see people watching out for each other – we're pack animals after all. To my mind, though, the most powerful tool to unite is sport. Meeting locals through joining a team can be a great remedy to loneliness. Most of my best friends in life have come from playing sports; it really does bring you closer to people. When you share the raw emotion that sport brings – joy, excitement, frustration, disappointment – it's so bonding. For a lot of people, sport also offers an escape. It allows you to express yourself, vent frustration and put life on the backburner for a bit.

And for those of you wanting a bit of time out (or time in, depending on how you look at it), there are disciplines here that are the bomb whether practised in groups or alone, depending on how you're feeling. Sometimes you might be up for joining the masses at your local Parkrun or dropping into a midweek yoga class after work, while at other times a 15-minute YouTube stretching session before work will be just the ticket. The beauty with these is that you can fit them around your life. Get away from your desk at lunchtime and do a 5k – it'll keep you so much more focused for an afternoon of work than a questionable coffee from your office drinks machine.

What's happening in there?

Remember the energy systems I explained earlier? This is where knowing a little about these comes in handy, because it means you can identify your exercise of choice along with an understanding of what's required on the body. Most exercise will use a combination of systems, with one being predominant. Here's a little recap:

Anaerobic Alactic (ATP-CP): This is all about short, efficient bursts of energy and is the predominant system at use for weightlifting, sprinting and gymnastics.

Anaerobic Lactic (glycolytic): This is for medium to high levels of intensity, and has a higher capacity than the ATP-CP system. Footballers and runners harness this system.

Aerobic: This one is all about the oxygen, so essential for activities based on continuous exertion and high levels of endurance. If long-distance swimming or rowing are your thing, this is the system in your body you'll want to be focusing on.

If you're not quite sure which system the training you're doing, or are about to start, is working, keep in mind that if you raise your heart rate over its normal resting rate for a sustained period of time, you're doing cardio. Cardiac hypertrophy, which is the thickening of the heart muscle, means the heart grows bigger and the stroke volume (this is the amount of blood pumped from the left ventricle) increases during exercise. Strengthening your heart makes it more efficient at pumping more blood per beat as your resting heart rate decreases.

Myth-busting

There is so much misinformation out there in the world of fitness, so I'm going to bust some of the big-gun myths. Fitness industry, please stop this madness!

Myth #1: You can target fat loss in your body

If there was a secret to this, we'd all know about it, so save your sanity and stop willing it to happen. Depending on your body type, genetic history, diet and lifestyle, you might have a tendency to gain fat in particular areas, such as the stomach, thighs or backside. This can naturally take a bit more effort to shift as we get older. While you can do exercises that target certain areas (like how sits-ups focus on the abs), you cannot disproportionately burn fat in one area. This is why women sometimes frustratingly find they might lose weight from an area they didn't want to, like the breasts, at the same time as the areas they *want* to lose it from, such as their middle.

Myth #2: Strength training is only for 'meatheads'

I wish this was old news, but it's something I often still hear. Listen out – everyone who is able should be doing some resistance training several times a week. I listed the benefits of strength training on page 77, and this is the case whether you are lifting weights or using your body weight as resistance. If you're worried about getting too bulky doing compound exercises like squats and lifting dumbbells, don't be – you have to train in a very deliberate way to make those kinds of gains!

Myth #3: On the subject of resistance training, not everything counts as 'resistance'

If you've ever been to a gym, you may have seen those tiddly little biscuit weights, i.e. the smallest plates on the planet, which are 1.25kg. So now imagine people using objects that are a fraction of that weight – toilet roll, teddies, cushions, which weigh only 100–350g – as 'resistance'. The world is full of people doing this and I don't know why! It's embarrassing. I'm actually mortified for them.

Myth #4: Functional madness

Functional training, in principle, is a really useful approach – it is a way of exercising that builds core muscles in the body, which in turn helps people with normal daily movement. But some (I blame the internet) have taken it to pointless extremes, adding ineffectual bits of kit like resistance bands and even blindfolds, kidding themselves it ramps up the training. Stop taking the clickbait piss. And for the record, you look possessed. I'll be sending cease-and-desist letters to the worst offenders.

Myth #5: Cardio training is the biggest calorie burner

Aerobic exercise can be a great way to burn calories and lose weight, but it's certainly not the only way. You may not be sweating buckets after a strength-training session, but depending on exactly what you're doing, there is potential to burn a shed load of calories – and you keep burning them after your workout.

Myth #6: The scales don't lie

Ah, but they do. Scales don't differentiate between fat and muscle mass (the latter of which is more dense), they don't know what time of day it is (we are generally lighter when we wake up, before we've eaten anything) or about water weight (when we eat certain foods, such as those that contain carbohydrates, they are stored in the body alongside a corresponding amount of water). Scales aren't useless, but they only give you a part of the picture.

JUMP

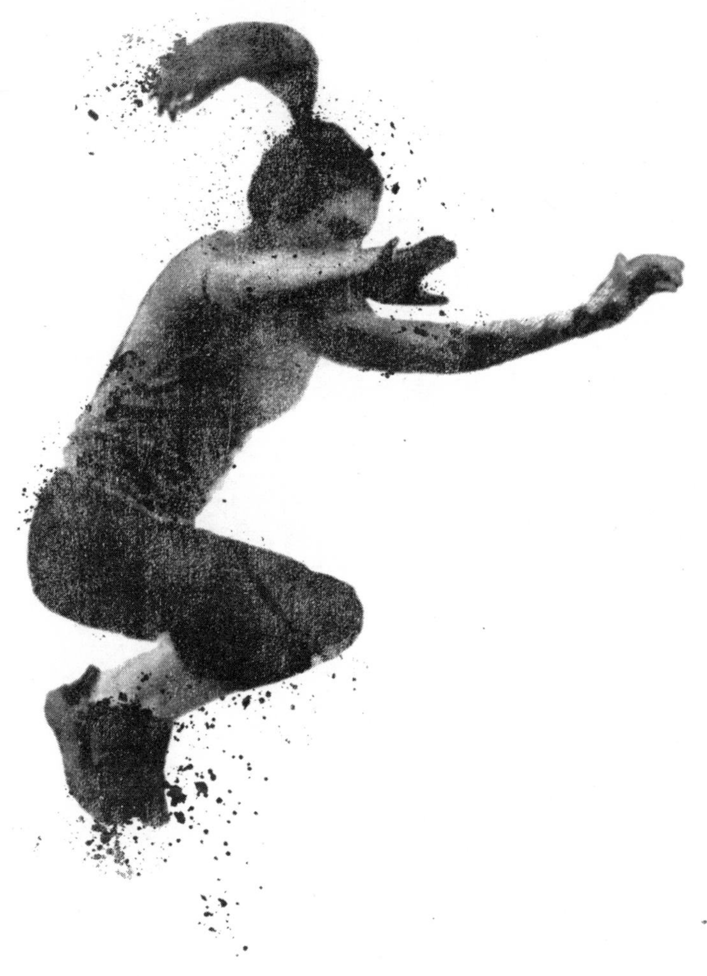

JUMP IS ALL about fitness that builds either from explosive movements and agility (as with HIIT and plyometrics), endurance (such as running) or a combination of all of those (as with boxing). Incorporating cardio-based training and doing movements like these on a regular basis trains the body to increase blood flow to the muscles, improving their ability to draw on oxygen and become more efficient. In the previous section, we looked at how the cardio and respiratory systems deliver oxygen around body and how training strengthens these systems. Essentially, you get an increase in lung capacity as you are able to hold more oxygen inside them, and this is what helps you become fitter. For example, the first time you try a rowing machine, at the start you'll be out of breath, but you then get stronger, your body adapts and develops, so it takes more to knacker you. And by the way, while it isn't one of the training regimes here, using a rowing machine at the gym is a brilliant whole-body workout, and one of the ultimate ways to build cardio fitness.

Give this type of training a whirl if you're looking for a challenge – just remember to check in first with your GP before embarking on any new fitness regime.

CROSSFIT AND HIIT

> 'I love CrossFit because it's diverse and challenging – you need to be good at so many different elements of fitness. The CrossFit community is really special too; you end up training alongside close friends, so there's an amazing atmosphere.'
>
> ZACK GEORGE, CROSSFIT GAMES COMPETITOR AND UK'S FITTEST MAN 2020

CrossFit is a relatively recent style of workout that involves high-intensity interval training that focuses on strength and core conditioning to build overall power, speed, endurance and agility. It uses equipment as well as your own body weight, and one of the many positives of CrossFit is that it's accessible for any level, because you can vary the intensity depending on your capability.

As the name suggests, several components of fitness are incorporated in CrossFit, including aerobic endurance, metabolic conditioning, elements of gymnastics, as well as weightlifting. I've done some training with Zack George (not that I could keep up with him) and at his elite level the training is intense AF. Zack trains two or three times a day (yes, I've written that correctly), for two hours each time, six days a week. During his one 'rest' day, there's no sofa lounging or cuddling up with a Deliveroo and Netflix (two of my best friends) – it's an active recovery day, so he goes swimming. CrossFit is one of the most mentally challenging exercises I've ever done.

Were I to ask a CrossFitter if they're a wolf or bear, they'd get to respond with a very smug 'both', because CrossFit is a discipline that prizes a whole-body approach. CrossFitters hold the reputation as being the fittest people in the world – a nice accolade, that's for sure. Whatever you throw at them is like water off a duck's back: climbing a wall, walking on their hands, running through sand – they're likely to nail it, so its broad spectrum makes it a pretty amazing discipline. In this training, you'll learn to mobilise your body and to use it in different ways. When CrossFit first became a thing, bodybuilders used laugh at them and take the piss (some still do!), but I reckon that's because they were jealous of how well CrossFitters can move across different plains. I wouldn't find it something to laugh at – in fact it's the opposite: the thought of training with Zack again makes me want to curl up in a corner and cry.

CrossFitters may not be as strong as a seasoned powerlifter or have the same endurance as a long-distance runner, but they'd give both strength training and cardio a very respectable shot. In short, they're the kings and queens of fitness. CrossFit is a high-impact sport and, for that reason, if you're reaching advanced levels it mightn't be a discipline you can sustain indefinitely.

How to do CrossFit

The way to train is to go to a CrossFit gym and learn the moves there, using the specialist equipment under the guidance of expert trainers. Most of these gyms will let you come and try a class for free, so go along and see what you think. Each workout you follow is scaled, so everyone does the same one but in varying degrees of difficulty depending on ability. In practice, this means that if you're new to CrossFit, you'll follow the weightlifting workout along with everyone else, but you'll lift less heavy weights and possibly for a shorter amount of time. Then you gradually scale it up as you become stronger.

The classes you attend at a CrossFit gym will focus on the different elements of the sport, mixing them up so that you, in turn, alternate the muscle groups used and give them a chance to adequately recover.

CrossFit competitions

Of course, you can train for CrossFit without giving two hoots about the competitive element, but I've known people who start training just for fun or as a way to get super-fit, and then get hooked and start competing. There are loads of competitions all over the world and many of them are tailored for people of all abilities, not just elite level. Competitions include rounds that test your cardio strength, weightlifting power and endurance. You might be swimming in the sea one minute and scaling a wall the next.

Watch any of these events on TV, such as the CrossFit Games, and it might make you want to leap out of your chair to try a bit of walking on your hands (looks cool/weird, I know). You'll notice a lot of people's surnames end in 'son' or 'dotter', and that's because CrossFit is hugely popular in countries like Iceland. They can't get enough. If it all goes tits up with powerlifting, I'll move to Reykjavík, change my name to Paul Olimasson and strive to be a CrossFit champ.

Mind how you go

In terms of safety and longevity, I do think there are elements of CrossFit to be wary about. I'd question whether some of the weightlifting elements of CrossFit – the ones that draw on movements from other disciplines, such as the Olympic lifting ones (the deadlift and the clean and presses, for example) – are designed for endurance. This is what happens when they're applied to CrossFit, where you'll sometimes have to complete, say, twelve clean and presses in a row (in some competitions it might be more). Other rounds might challenge you to do as many deadlifts as you can in an allotted timeframe. Naturally, when you're bashing out that kind of high number, you'll become exhausted, and as a result your form and positioning, as well as your focus, can easily slip. Good technique just can't be sustained, so it can be really dangerous, especially when you're moving such heavy weights. There are some exercises out there that just aren't designed to be endurance sports. Are these included in CrossFit competitions just to add another element of extreme sport? I wonder if that's the case. There's no doubt it's awe inspiring to watch a CrossFitter at their peak, but the weight categories raise some alarm bells with me, so I'd advise you to approach with caution. There's a high rate of injury in this sport, so remember to listen to your body and not overdo it.

High-intensity interval training (HIIT)

> 'HIIT is a great way to exercise. No equipment or large space is required – the perfect way to kick-start your day.'
>
> BRADLEY SIMMONDS, KING OF HIIT

I wanted to cover HIIT here as it has become super-popular over recent years, and its appeal has only been boosted further by the most famous PE teacher in the world, the shiny-maned stallion Joe Wicks. Hats off to Joe for getting kids to move, especially during lockdown.

There's some crossover between HIIT and CrossFit in that they're both whole-body, fast-and-furious-style workouts that alternate between strength conditioning, using body weight (and sometimes free weights) as resistance, and aerobic drills. As with plyometric training, some sets also involve explosive movement. It's a great option if you're time-poor or if you're easily bored (you don't really have time to lose interest!), because it switches up the exercise so frequently. It works because it challenges the body's different energy systems, pushing the lactate system and working aerobically (see page 72). How long you do a HIIT session for (i.e. the time you are exercising versus the time you are resting in between) really varies depending on the regime you follow. It's these rest periods that are a key component of high-intensity training, varying from anything like 15 seconds to a minute or two (turn to page 197 where I talk about the value of strategic rest). Do not – I repeat, *do not* – skip them. They're as important as the exercises themselves, as they facilitate recovery as well as enabling you to re-energise for the next high-intensity burst. It's the short, sharp force of HIIT that keeps your body burning calories for the rest of the day, unlike other, less fast-paced aerobics workouts, such as going for a jog. In my opinion, some popular HIIT workouts don't factor in enough rest time, often only 30 seconds of rest after 30 seconds or more of exercise. The problem with this is that more rest is needed to tap into the anaerobic system.

HIIT can be done at the gym (either in a class or on the gym floor if there's space), at the park or at home, and you can start gradually to build up your strength and stamina, beginning with five or ten minutes if you're a total beginner. You can play around with the rest times too; just remember that the less rest you have in between, the more cardio-based your workout becomes, and when the rest periods are a bit longer, it becomes more about muscle-building. During the exercises, it's all about short bursts of high energy and really pushing yourself to give it your all, rather than doing slower drills over a longer period. So, get in and get out. All you really need equipment-wise is your regular sportswear; a mat is helpful for the core exercises you lie on your back for, but a towel is the next best thing. It's also a great discipline to try with friends, whether you're in a class together or doing the DIY route. I always find that training with friends spurs me on to push myself harder, if only to beat them (competitive? Me?). Get your trainers on, head to the park and set up a stopwatch (use your phone) to alternate between 'move' and 'rest'. Choose any number of combinations of the below for a 30-minute workout, and as you progress and get fitter, the intensity you do these at will naturally accelerate:

Whole-body: running on the spot, jumping jacks, ski steps, burpees, shuffle jumps, toe-touches, boxing punches, ladder drills (where special sports ladders are placed on the ground and you run through the gaps, challenging your agility), cone drills.

Legs: squats or squat jumps, lunges or jumping lunges (remember to do both legs), high knees, side lunges, duck walks, gorilla walks, bear walks, squat holds.

Arms: push-ups (if you can't do a full one, drop down to your knees), shoulder taps.

Core: plank, mountain climbers, Russian twists, sit-ups with legs extended or at a 90° angle, criss-cross legs, roll-down planks, butterfly crunches, squat thrusts, side planks (both sides).

HIIT and different fitness levels

If you're currently very unfit or overweight, some of the movements of HIIT might be more challenging. This type of training is a big ask for the body because the whole premise is based on maximal-effort movements in a short space of time, with some explosive, high-power movements thrown in there for good measure. Don't let this put you off, though, as there are modifications you can introduce, helping you to adapt HIIT to your ability. It can be really frustrating to be told (by trainers like myself!) in a blasé way to bash out 30 seconds of mountain climbers when, in reality, if you have a larger stomach, the mechanics of doing even one might be a no-go. So, for example, instead of doing a mountain climber, you might just have to hold the plank position (with knees on the floor if you can't hold them up). When you gradually start feeling more confident and mobile, try bringing one knee slowly into the stomach and back out again, swapping legs. You might also feel self-conscious attending class if you're less experienced, and worried you won't be able to keep up. To this I'd say, try not to let these worries hold you back – we all have our insecurities and, by and large, most people at the gym are focusing on their own development rather than being distracted by anyone else.

That being said, if you can't face doing a group workout, no problem, because a HIIT session in the privacy of your living room is totally doable.

Adapting exercises will help give you better form as well as reducing the risk of injury and putting pressure on your joints. HIIT is a very efficient workout if burning fat is your goal, and provided you ease into it, listen to your body and respect that getting fit and losing weight is a process rather than a quick fix to be rushed, high-intensity exercises can be really effective. But, like anyone, you should always check in first with your GP before starting an exercise regime, especially if you've never done one before.

Top tips for adapting HIIT

Go at your own pace: HIIT tends to be harder the less fit and nimble you are, and it's more challenging if you're carrying extra weight because this restricts your mobility. For example, it's trickier leaping up and down off the floor doing a burpee if you can't sustain more than one. In the long run, as you get fitter, the intensity will increase, but in the meantime, do what you can while still getting a sweat on. Lots of exercises can be carried out at a more moderate pace (e.g. star jumps can be done one side at a time, with one foot always on the floor), so look for ways to slow it down if you need to.

Embrace exercises in line with your range of motion: Certain positions require greater mobility (such as the ones where you need to lift your body up off the floor), but there are plenty of others you can do – things like half jacks, stepping-back jacks, reverse lunges, leg extensions, hamstring curls, diagonal jacks, standing tree pose (using the wall for balance if you need to), leg circles (lying with your back on the mat), standing push-ups (against a wall). There are many, many more out there; I'd go as far as to say that most of them can be tailored to your own personal level of fitness and mobility.

Consider bringing in some added resistance: The list of HIIT exercises I gave a little earlier all use body weight to build strength, but there are lots of HIIT fans out there, of all abilities, who like to incorporate weights such as dumbbells (which you can buy relatively cheaply). Often people carrying extra weight are pretty strong and powerful, and increasing the intensity this way is a better option than ramping up the cardio aspect.

Revisit and reassess: You may not be able to manage a set of push-ups right now, but if you keep training, you will be. So, check in every week or two to revisit any exercises you haven't been able to do and give them another go – you never know! It might take a little while to manage a set of squat thrusts, but you'll get there, and when you do, it means you can start incorporating these once-elusive movements into your routine.

CROSSFIT AND HIIT

What CrossFit and HIIT delivers: With CrossFit, you'll be the fittest person you can be. Even if you already train and feel fit, CrossFit will take it to another level. HIIT delivers a time-efficient workout that gives bang for its buck.

Why they work: They provide a whole-body workout that brings in both cardio and strength elements.

Physique: Part wolf, part bear – need I say more?

Pros: You'll have both aerobic fitness as well as strength (muscular upper and lower body) – strong but agile and athletic.

Cons: Injury is common in CrossFit as it's very demanding and easy to overdo.

Equipment: HIIT can be done using just your body weight as resistance but CrossFit uses kit such as kettlebells, battle ropes, sandbags, jumping boxes – the list goes on.

Importance of technique: With CrossFit there's a lot to learn, particularly with the weightlifting categories; time must be spent perfecting positions such as the deadlift and the overhead press. If your form is off, it makes injury much more likely.

BOXING

> 'Boxing is a great workout because it challenges you both physically and mentally. It takes tremendous concentration and focus – it's like playing chess while running on a treadmill. It's been proven that when you really concentrate on training, you burn more calories.'
>
> ANTHONY YARDE, WORLD LIGHT HEAVYWEIGHT CONTENDER

Put simply, boxing is the art of hitting and not getting hit. Although from the outside it may look like a blood sport, it really is an artform; there's a grace in the movements and rhythm of the pros. When doing research for this book, I caught up with my so-called mate Anthony Yarde. I hopped into the ring with him so that he could put me through my paces. He ended up beating seven shades of shite out of me. Some friend.

I've always had an interest in boxing and have massive respect for boxers who not only combine cardio fitness with serious power but who are also all about discipline and mental strength. It's one of the very best sports you can do if you're looking for an all-round workout, as it conditions every muscle group. And it's fun! Above all other benefits, for me this one is the most important. So I had to include boxing here.

It's also a banging spectator sport and I often go to watch fights. Watching someone like Anthony Joshua in the ring is a spectacle. The atmosphere and love for him from the crowd is always electric. I've body-doubled for him (though he's definitely taller than me!), and he's such a lovely guy, but when you see him fearlessly attacking his opponent in the ring (fluids flying every which way!), you see the warhorse – gloves on, total focus.

When I was about fifteen, I trained at a local club in Blanchardstown in Dublin for six months or so. At that stage I was playing in the top schoolboy football league and was well used to training several times a week. I had all the energy of a hyper teenager and could run endlessly. So, I got a shock when I started boxing and I couldn't even last three rounds – my body just couldn't cope with the demands that kind of exercise was throwing at it – speed, agility, endurance and explosive power – and all required simultaneously. It was the same when, later in life, I started Brazilian Jiu Jitsu and wrestling; after rolling around for a few minutes on the mat, I was gone. Forget lifting weights or kicking a ball about – martial arts training is the most challenging thing I've ever done.

Again, I returned to boxing and mixed martial arts after I'd stopped playing football and was wondering what to do next. I wanted to keep my fitness up and give myself another challenge after years of running – training and gym work. I was taken by surprise yet again by how unprepared I was for the crazy demands of this type of sport. I was having a go at something like wrestling but would be hung out to dry after a few minutes of grappling and being held down. Keeping at it, my body did adapt, and of course it helped that I had a great base level of fitness from having played football and hitting the weights. But seriously, it pushed me to my max. Massive respect to anyone who trains in this way – you're a beast.

I want to emphasise, and this should go without saying, that boxing is an equally brilliant sport for women, though of course, unfairly, professional boxing is dominated by male fighters. This means that for many women it may not necessarily cross their minds as a fitness option. Rest assured, there are more women pulling the gloves on, and astonishingly skilled boxers like Nicola Adams and Katie Taylor are inspiring a new generation of women into the ring.

Boxing clever

Boxing (and all martial arts) draws on significant mental focus – when you're sparring, you can't let your mind wander for a second (unless you fancy peeling your sweaty face off the ring floor after you've been knocked out). Your motor skills get a workout too, as your hand–eye coordination develops every time you punch. And if you need any more convincing that boxing is the ultimate workout: if ever there was a stress-reliever, this is it. Take your bad mood out on the punch bag and you'll feel like a new person after your session, as the endorphins kick in. It's the best way that I know of to relieve frustration or pent-up energy. Even the most aggressive individual is as calm as a lamb after a workout.

Boxing can be a real wake-up call too, highlighting any dodgy habits. Most people find that once they start boxing, it really dawns on them how amazing their body is, because it responds quickly to this type of workout. On day one, your punch might be slow, but skedaddle two weeks and it'll be a different story. If you catch the bug, at each session you'll want to be that bit stronger, that bit more agile and powerful than you were at the last one. These speedy progressions make you want to look after your body by eating well and generally behaving yourself a bit more! It's not uncommon for people with a dicey past, whether that involves drugs, booze, smoking or junk food, to find that boxing makes them want to ditch the old habits.

Training

Much of the training in a gym involves hitting pads and hitting a bag. It's a high-energy, high-calorie-burning workout. You'll be focusing on developing your technique for the four main punches – the jab, the hook, the uppercut and the cross – as well as footwork and stances. In addition to developing these specific skills, you'll be ramping up the overall fitness needed to box. And it's hardcore because it draws on all your energy systems (aerobic, anaerobic and lactate systems), which is why boxing is considered a 'complete' workout: cardio, strength conditioning, explosive movements and stamina – if you get into the training, your fitness levels will soar.

The level of involvement with boxing can be as much or as little as you want, so you set the pace of what you want to do – whether that's training alone doing shadow boxing in front of your bedroom mirror, skipping and running or going all in, joining a boxing gym and competing in organised amateur fights. You can decide how far you want to go and it's this flexibility that's another reason I love it.

If you decide to join a club, you'll be taught the principles of boxing – the punches, defence movements, stances, footwork and how to conjure mental strength and focus. At a club, before you start sparring, you'll also watch and learn a lot. Observing boxers of all levels training can be really inspiring – you'll see what and what not to do, and there's the all-important social element. When you do start sparring, you'll probably feel a bit nervous and self-conscious, as it feels like a big step up from laying into the bag. Take your frenemy with you and you'll get to punch him or her in the face, no questions asked. Another bonus of boxing.

If you've been sparring for a while at your boxing gym, you might want to start competing in amateur matches against people of similar levels from other stables. The next stage would be to turn professional (when you go pro, you can't return to amateur).

If you don't fancy going to a boxing gym, most regular gyms run fitness classes which are based around boxing moves, and have both aerobic and strength elements. These sessions can give a great introduction to the sport and an insight into the type of training involved. There you'll likely be partnered up to punch and block and take it in turns to hold the bag, as well as doing a variety of other drills to challenge your fitness. These classes are usually suitable for total beginners, so you don't need to feel sheepish about being a newbie – and you won't get hit (not on day one anyway!). You might go to one class a week as part of your wider routine or go hell for leather and make boxing your passion, doing it a few times each week.

Again, if that sounds too involved and you want to hit at neither a boxing club nor a commercial gym, or there are none near you, you can set up your own DIY Fight Club (minus the bare knuckles and fag in your mouth) at home. You can shadow box or, even better, hang a bag wherever you have the space and start playing around, throwing punches and practising your footwork.

Boxing workout

Here's a taster of a boxing training session and a decent work-out you can try yourself in the gym (or at home if you have the gear). Don't be afraid of getting punched – you're not made of glass and once you take a couple of jabs, you'll realise it's not that bad and it doesn't hurt as much as you think it will! Your boxing coach will match you appropriately with another boxer.

Running: To keep up aerobic fitness, running short to medium distances is a standard part of boxing training. When you do a 5k run as a boxer, you're doing it to make you stronger in the ring. Knowing that the run will enable you to swing punches for longer and improve your endurance when you are sparring will make even the most running-phobic (me!) motivated to pound the pavement. So, for the first part of the workout, follow the dynamic warm-ups (see page 129) and then do a 4–5k run at a fair pace.

Conditioning and core strength work (10 sets of 2–3 minutes, with 30 seconds of rest, for each of the below):

- Medicine ball: There are lots of drills you can do with a medicine ball (a weighted ball, which is a common bit of kit used in resistance training and will be found in most, if not all, gyms), but one simple one is simply throwing one back and forth with a pal. If you stand slightly further apart than comfortable, you'll be working harder.
- Sit-ups
- Skipping
- Shadow boxing

Jump rope (5 sets of 2–3 minutes): This is a brilliant exercise to aid balance and coordination as it helps the body get used to hopping weight between the right and left side, a rhythm which is integral to sparring. There's no hanging about in boxing; you're always on the move. It may not look particularly dynamic, but jump rope challenges muscles in the whole body and is harder than it looks, so if you can't manage five rounds, just do what you can and gradually build it up each session.

Heavy bag (5 rounds of 2–3 minutes): Another high-intensity drill that will help condition the upper body and core by burning fat and building muscle.

Sparring (2–3-minute rounds or as many as you want – usually 3–4, depending on your level): You'll typically end a session sparring with someone (or shadow boxing if you're solo), putting into practice any moves you've covered in the session (particularly any new ones). This is about developing technique rather than going all out, so pay attention to each move, going more slowly if you need to in order to improve your delivery. Sparring is the ultimate test of fitness.

Stretches to **cool down:**

Hamstrings: Begin by standing upright, feet together and firmly planted on the floor. Bend over, reaching your hands down to touch your toes.

Quads: With one foot planted firmly on the ground, bend the other knee and kick your foot back towards your backside, using your hand to hold it here (you may need to hold onto a wall for balance). After you feel a good stretch, repeat on the other side.

Shoulders: Standing up, stretch your right arm out and bring your left hand just above your right elbow. Pull the right arm so that you feel a good stretch. Repeat on the other side.

Triceps: Standing straight with feet hip-width apart,

stretch the right arm up to the ceiling, bend the elbow and reach the right hand down between your shoulder blades. Place the left hand on the right elbow, gently pressing the elbow down. Repeat on the other side.

BOXING

What boxing delivers: Strength, stamina and agility as well as a mental workout. View it as the works.

Why it works: It's an incredible full-body workout.

Physique: You'll lean up, probably losing body fat and getting into your 'fighting weight'. You'll be light on your feet too ('float like a butterfly, sting like a bee' etc.).

Pros: You'll be strong all over, and it improves balance and coordination. It's a stress-buster, and you'll learn key self-defence moves should you ever need to protect yourself inside or outside of the ring.

Cons: If you're competing, you're likely to get a beating (unless you're Floyd Mayweather).

Equipment: Padded gloves, face guard, gum shield, boots, hand wraps.

Importance of technique: You'll learn the stances and positions as well as punches and blocks.

RUNNING

When I look back at all the years I played football, it's the running element I remember most. (I'm pretty sure we all used to call it jogging – when did 'running' become a thing for amateurs?) In Ireland we had some inspiring runners too, who dazzled on the screen when I was growing up. Sonia O'Sullivan was a national hero, setting records at the time and bringing home an Olympic medal in 2000. Even now, watching athletics, particularly at the Olympics and Paralympics, is a highlight – from the excitement of sprinting to witnessing the unbelievable endurance of marathon runners and wheelchair racers; it's exhilarating stuff.

Can I do a bit of running-related name-dropping now please? When I used to work as a body double, one happy day I got a call asking if I could double up for an athlete I'd never worked with before. Their usual double wasn't available so they needed a stand-in. By this point, I'd been doing this type of work (though it never really felt like work) for a few years, and through a bit of right-time-right-place luck, I had carved out a niche stepping in for the most prominent male, Black athletes around. *Yeah, yeah, yeah, get to the bleedin' point*, I hear you shouting. Okay, it was Usain Bolt. *Usain. Bolt.* This man I'd watched on telly speed over the finish line, pushing the boundaries of sport, with me and the rest of the world copying his lightning bolt pose. Here he was singing and dancing on set. I remember looking down and noticing his Achilles tendon, which was absolutely *mahooosive*. It looked bigger than my whole calf! I've never seen anything like it. I'm pretty sure it must be the secret to his record-setting.

Anyhoo, I reckon the surge in the popularity of running must be in part down to the pros inspiring us. While it also forms the basis of the training for many other cardio-based sports, especially those which rely on endurance, needless to say it's an activity in itself. Just head to a park on a Saturday morning, anywhere from Eswatini to Japan, and you'll see a pack of enthusiasts sweating their way through a Parkrun. It's funny to think that going out for a jog only really became a 'thing' in the 1960s and '70s. Before then, if you'd donned your shorts for a gallop around the green, people would have gawked at you like you'd lost your mind.

Some people love running in the great outdoors with different terrains challenging the leg muscles, while others prefer the treadmill, which is easier on the legs. You don't need a gym membership or a personal trainer (or even shoes, if you fancy being one of those barefoot jogging types ... think I'll keep my trainers on, thanks). It's easy to fit in around life, especially if you're doing shorter or mid-length runs; you can do it close to home or on holidays if you want to keep up a bit of fitness, and if you work somewhere where there are showers, it can also be a great option for a lunch-time excursion. Unlike some other types of exercise, even ones covered in this book, you can get started now – as in right *now*. Yes, there are different theories and training practices for running, but in the first instance you could always just have a go – you know what to do: put one foot after the other in a straight-ish line – and see how you get on. After a few initial runs, you can begin to focus more on technique and posture, as in the long run (*ba-boom*), the mechanics of how you run will help prevent injury and improve your performance. If you're a total beginner who doesn't have much fitness, one trick is to just run for as long as you can (it might only be ten seconds) and then walk for the same amount of time. Keep alternating between running and walking, doing a roughly equal number of seconds and minutes of each. If you start running around three times a week, you will notice that every couple of runs, your endurance will have developed. One of the gratifying aspects of running is that you don't have to wait long to see results, particularly if you're new. You'll also start enjoying it more as you get better – it's hard to like something when it makes you feel like you're having a heart attack, I know, but give it a fair shot. And if you get into it and fancy a challenge to work towards, there have never been more events you can sign up to: 5ks, 10ks, half-marathons, marathons, ultramarathons – you'll have no trouble finding a race to suit you. A lot of people get the competitive running bug and start using events as an excuse for a holiday. *Copenhagen marathon? Why not! 10k in Rio? Don't mind if I do.* Plus, if you're training for longer races, it's a great excuse to get away from housemates or family if you need a break (or is that just me?).

Running is an activity you can enjoy in solitude (more on that coming up) or as a social exertion. Running clubs are a brilliant way to meet people and you don't necessarily have to be super-fast to join one, as many cater for all levels. Or you could even start your own informal one – I know of someone who put a poster up on her street saying that two evenings a week she'd be running a 5k and would start outside the corner shop at 7 p.m. if anyone wanted to join her. Before long the world and his wife were coming along, neighbours of all ability levels who'd change into their running kit after coming home from work, head to the corner shop and jog round the neighbourhood, chatting away as they did so. Bring your dog, bring your kid, bring your friend (or let them cycle beside you as a sergeant major shouting something motivational or abusive, depending on what incentivises you).

Walking

While we're on a similar subject, let's hear it for walking – the OG of exercise. Walking, briskly if possible, cannot be underestimated. It's why, funnily enough, you might be doing more for your body when you walk to the gym than you are when you're actually in the gym. Non-exercise activity thermogenesis (NEAT) is the term that describes the movement you do and the calories you burn when you aren't deliberately exercising. Walking up and down the stairs, doing household chores and strolling to the Tube station are all examples. And they can really add up, especially if you do a job that has you on your feet a lot.

Walking is often the first thing I recommend for people who are really out of shape or who are particularly intimidated by the prospect of getting fit (I can see the fear in their eyes). It's something you can build up slowly, literally going at a snail's pace at the start if you need to. Stick on some sunglasses if you enjoy incognito vibes, lash the earphones in and away you go.

> 'Walking is something we should be doing on a daily basis, both for energy expenditure and also for the mental benefits as we put ourselves in different environments. There's so much to see in this world and one of the best ways to do so is by walking and exploring – have you ever noticed you get

those lightbulb moments while walking? Allowing your body to wander will impact your mental health more than you know. Stay moving. It keeps us alive.'

DIREN KARTAL, CREATOR OF #NEATUP247

Running to clear your head

A bit of headspace is a wonderful thing, and that's what you'll get when you head out on a jog. Just had a blazing row with your partner? Go out for a run. Been cooped up in the office all day? Go out for a run. Need some time to gather your thoughts? You've guessed it – God, you're smart – go out for a run. Catching up with a friend while running is nice, but so is alone time. Many people testify to the meditative tonic that comes with pounding the pavement. Some say that's when they have their best ideas; others say they have no ideas (and for them, that's the point – they switch off).

I've never had much time for the treadmill, and when I used to run, back in the days when I could do laps for hours and not get tired, it was always outdoors. If machine running is your pleasure, by all means go for it. For many people, it's being outside that adds to the mental health benefits – getting some daylight and a bit of vitamin D if the sun's out, seeing some greenery if you're in a park, running along a beach or perhaps being in a rural setting (not that I'd know the front end of a cow from the back). Even if you live in a concrete jungle, it can feel a bit more freeing than running in a gym (maybe not if it's pissing down with rain though).

Keep the form

Your position when you run is really important, as it affects your performance and helps to keep your energy expenditure efficient, meaning you'll tire less quickly. It can also prevent injury, as well as minimising aches and pains after a run. If you are prone to injury, particularly in the knee joints, or worried about getting one, check out chi running. It brings in some principles from tai chi and yoga and focuses on preventing injuries by running in a way that is as low impact as possible as well as paying close attention to alignment.

Adjusting your mechanics might feel a bit unnatural at first, but before long you'll start noticing that the tweaks pay off. So, after you've done a few runs, start thinking about posture, incorporating the following techniques, in order to avoid injury.

Upper body: Often when you see someone out jogging their upper body is too far forwards, as if something is pushing their shoulders towards the ground. It means their core isn't engaged and so the lower back isn't protected. The upper body should propel forwards a little, so there's no need to keep it dead vertical, but you should be lengthening through your spine rather than slumping.

Shoulders and arms: It's common to default to hunching your shoulders as you run, but keep them down, drawing them back a bit so that your shoulder blades feel activated. Maintaining a broad chest will help with your shoulder positioning. Your elbows should stay close to your body when you're running and bent at a roughly 90° angle. Think about Mr Tickle's arms lolloping down aimlessly – this is what you *don't* want happening! Keep your arms coordinated, swinging rhythmically with your legs when in motion. Your hands should be in a loose fist.

Core: Imagine there's an invisible band around your waist propelling you forward, with your pelvis very slightly lifted – keep this visual in mind and let a lot of your force be driven from this area. If you keep focused on this, it'll not only help you to keep your core activated, but it can help prevent your back's position from slipping. Your hips should be positioned over the middle of your feet, helping to stabilise the pelvis and keeping the key leg muscles engaged.

Legs and knees: Good knee alignment can help maintain your body's optimum positioning and work towards keeping the dreaded runner's knee at bay. Keep the knees parallel and activated so that they don't cave in. Try to land gently rather than hammering the pavement like you hate your feet. With this in mind, many people find that running on grassy surfaces, rather than hard, concrete ones, gives less knee and foot pain after a run. Wearing good-quality running shoes will also help your alignment.

Feet: Lift those feet! I don't mean you need to be doing high knees with every stride (you'd be knackered pretty quickly), but dragging them on the ground (which often happens towards the end of a run when you're tired) is not a friend to overall form and is a big trip hazard. Maintain good alignment by keeping your feet hip-width apart. Aim to land each stride on the middle of your foot, avoiding your toes and heels, and maintaining balance. You should invest in a good pair of trainers, fitted by an expert, that support all the bones in your feet as well as your ankles. Staff in sports shops, particularly in running-specific stores, are trained to assess your gait and will ask about the type of running you do as well as the frequency so that they can match you to your perfect kicks. I remember the first time I brought proper running shoes (rather than just general trainers not specifically designed for running) with orthopaedic soles – it was life-changing, especially because I have quite flat feet, so the extra support felt amazing.

How to train for running

Yes, you can just run around the park as normal, but if you do want to push yourself to improve speed and/or endurance or if you are training for a race (or even just to save your sanity, in case you're getting bored), it's a good idea to diversify your routine. If you're into running as your main exercise and you go several times a week, a simple way to shake up your training would be to allocate a different strand of training to each session. So, if you run three times a week, one run would focus on improving speed (fartlek training), another run would be all about building endurance (the low and slow technique) and being able to run further, and your third run might focus on recovery, regenerating strength for you to do it all again the following week. It's the combination of these different styles that leads to gains. Here are some popular training methods that can be applied, scaling up or down, for any ability.

Fartlek training

This is based on the principal of varying the type of training, frequently altering the speed at which you run, the distance and even the terrain underfoot, so that you keep progressing, getting faster and increasing endurance. It's easy in running to reach a plateau, especially if you are someone who does the same route and isn't particularly looking at the clock when it comes to your speed – which, by the way, is totally fine if you're happy with that approach. If you do want to keep developing though, playing around with the intensity of some of your runs will keep your body adapting. There are loads of ways you can do that, and it's best to mix up the techniques, but one really simple way to start is, on one of your weekly runs, break up a 30-minute session by alternating between sprinting (where you go full throttle) and jogging. Play around with timings, but one minute of jogging and 10 seconds of sprinting will give you a solid starting point, and as you progress you can increase the sprint length. There are apps that will facilitate the timings, sounding an alarm so that you know when to switch. If you're not used to this, you'll probably find it pretty tiring, as you'll be switching between energy systems (the aerobic and anaerobic) when you mix up the intensity. If you need to stop sprinting or jogging, that's okay, but try to keep walking if you can.

Variety training

A little like what Fartlek has to offer, adding a session a week where you change up some element of your run will help your body adapt, reaching those fast-twitch muscles and keeping stagnation at bay. High-intensity drills such as sprinting are a good way to do this, as is doing a shorter run each week, as part of your routine, but at a faster pace. There are also changes you can make to your environment that will help build speed. Hill running (which you can also do on a treadmill when it's set at an incline) or even running on different terrains will add a new dimension to your training. Another option is running with a weighted backpack, which I'm sure you've seen some runners wearing. This is to help build muscular endurance, by making you run harder; it'll also burn more calories. Don't just throw on your old school bag, though! You'll need a proper running backpack that you can add weights to and remove when you need to, that fits snugly and doesn't jiggle when you run. Carrying weight on your back will obviously make your job harder and puts more direct pressure on the shoulders and back. See how you get on with this, as it's not for everyone, and if you do try it, be sure to build up the weights gradually. You might find at the start you can't run quite as far as you can without the bag, but the body will adapt, and as it does, you can increase the weight if you like.

Low and slow

If you are looking to improve endurance, you'll likely be doing a longer run most weeks. Gradually elongating these runs is how you boost your overall capacity, so aim to add one or two minutes on each time and gradually go from there. Don't worry if you can't manage these extras minutes' running (time has a habit of slowing down for these) – dropping down to walk is okay. The idea with these longer runs is that you do them at a comfortable pace rather than 100%.

Recovery run

I mention a few times in this book how I've failed to listen to my body and given myself proper time to recover between training (whether that was when I played rugby or, more recently, when I lift at the gym). It's so tempting, especially when you feel like you're making good progress or you are training for an upcoming competition or race, to go bananas with the training. It's counter-intuitive but, believe me, in the long run it'll slow you down and hamper your gains if you don't give your body time to rest. So, if you're running several times a week, you need to include a recovery session. Depending on your level (i.e. how far you usually run), this will be a short- or medium-distance run – if you're a beginner it might only be a mile; if you're a proficient half-marathon runner, it might be more like five miles – do what's right for you. No matter the mileage covered, though, the idea is that you complete this run at a slow jog, keeping your heart rate low. It might feel weird and annoying going at a snail's pace, or you might think it's a waste of time – it's not. As well as helping with recovery, see it as giving your body a little MOT. Focus on each of your body parts, starting with your feet and going up through the ankles and calves, all the way up through your upper body too. Because you're not pushing yourself too hard, you'll notice any niggles, tightness or imbalances that might need addressing later through stretching, mobility work, massage or physio.

Warm-up and cool-down

I just love taking time for these. Said no one ever. But you do need to do both, despite what some people think. Make sure your warm-ups are dynamic (I've given an example below), rather than those puny stretches where you're basically stationary. Dynamic stretches send a signal to the central nervous system telling it to start firing up, so that mind and body are supporting you in your run. They'll also get the blood flowing and begin to mobilise the joints. Here's a straightforward warm-up to do before your run, whatever your level and the distance you're running. It only takes a few minutes and you don't need to rest in between these exercises; just motor through the warm-up and be gone. There are also some cool-down exercises to do afterwards.

Dynamic warm-up stretches

If you'd like to see these and other exercises in action, go to my website (www.theomegaarmy.com/workout-videos).

EXERCISE	***REPS***	***SETS***
Forward leg swings	10 on each side	1
Side leg swings	10 on each side	1
Opposite toe touches	10 on each side	1
High knees	30 seconds	1
Tuck jumps	30 seconds	1
Lateral run	30 seconds	1
Leaping bound	30 seconds	1
Single-leg heel tuck	30 seconds	1

Cool-down stretches

EXERCISE	***REPS***	***SETS***
Kneeling hip flexor stretch	20 seconds on each side	1
Seated calf stretch (use a resistance band if you have one)	20 seconds on each side	1
Standing hamstring stretch	20 seconds on each side	1
Reclined pigeon glute stretch	20 seconds on each side	1
Lunge groin stretches	20 seconds on each side	1
Side-lying quad stretch	20 seconds on each side	1
Knees-to-chest stretch for the lower back	30 seconds	1
Shoulder-opening stretch, holding onto a doorway for resistance and support	30 seconds	1

RUNNING

What running delivers: Cardiovascular fitness, endurance and stress release.

Why it works: It burns calories, tones the body and brings mental clarity by giving you the feeling of 'getting away from it all'.

Physique: This will vary a bit depending on the type you're doing (e.g. sprinting or longer distance), but if it's mid- to long-distance you can expect to be muscular and lean, and if it's shorter lengths you'll likely be bigger.

Pros: It can be a good option for losing weight. Many find it relaxing and, as your cardio fitness improves, you'll find everyday tasks easy-peasy. It's a great activity to do alone or with peeps.

Cons: Like most sports, there is a risk of injury and of overdoing it. A lot of running can be tough on the knee joints.

Equipment: You don't need a lot of kit to be a runner, but a decent pair of trainers are a must, as they will help support you. You can have these fitted by an expert if you go to a running shop. If you like listening to music or podcasts as you run, then those little arm pouches that you can clip your phone into are useful.

Measuring progress: Depending on the types of training, you'll be able to run further and/or faster.

Importance of technique: If you're running regularly, good technique, in the form of your body's running posture, is vital both to help you progress and to avoid injury.

PLYOMETRIC TRAINING

> 'Track and field has moulded me into everything I dreamed of being as a young kid. Strong, fast, and Olympian – training with no limits and achieving superhuman feats! It's amazing what athletics can help you become.'
>
> HARRY AIKINES-ARYEETEY, 100M GB OLYMPIAN

Jump higher, run faster, throw further, hit harder! The magic of incorporating plyometrics into your routine is that it'll make you better in any other sport you do. You might also have heard this called 'shock' or 'jump' training. It's a discipline in itself but, more typically, it forms a vital part of training in a variety of sports, with the goal of improving overall athleticism so that you excel in your other training. Top athletes across a wide range of disciplines, such as boxers, weightlifters and sprinters, will include some plyo training within their wider programmes, but you don't need to be an Olympian to benefit from this approach – it can be a great way to crank your fitness up a notch whatever level you're at. It's becoming more mainstream, too, as more fitness enthusiasts realise that adding some plyometrics to their routine can really boost it.

Plyometrics are forms of exercises that push your muscles to their maximum (or near-maximum) capacity in a very short space of time. It was created by the Russian scientist Yuri Verkhoshansky about fifty years ago, and it's all about explosive movements, challenging both the upper and lower body. The basic principle is that during this type of movement, muscles are being repeatedly and rapidly stretched and then contracted. And it's quality over quantity with this type of training. It's not something you'll be practising for hours; it's more a case of short bursts at high effort.

It's amazing to watch the pros do plyometrics. They're almost like dancers; the movements they zip through are so coordinated – fast, but graceful too. There are a lot of techniques to master and, be warned, you'll look like a bit of a goon the first few times, trying to get the hang of the moves, but who cares? I was all over the shop when I started out. Like everything new, it takes a bit of getting used to.

If you are a plyometrics beginner, be sure to start slowly, adding in exercises gradually to build up your range and stamina. It's high-impact, so if you go at it full throttle, without steadily laying the foundations, you risk damaging your joints, tendons and ligaments.

Injury prevention

Avoiding injury is one of the big draws for me about this type of training, especially as the bodybuilding and powerlifting that I do really pushes my body (admittedly sometimes past its comfort zone). Lifting heavy weights puts a lot of pressure on the joints, and I'm always mindful of doing what I can to make me less susceptible to damage. It's why I do a lot of plyometrics, as it's very effective for preventing injury by improving alignment and stability of key joints, like the hips, knees and ankles, through jumping movements and landing techniques. Simple exercises would include working on your posture and alignment, for example, so that when you jump, your knees are controlled and don't cave in, and your feet land together, 'sticking' (a plyo term) and not leaning forward. Poor knee alignment means your body is not being fully supported, and that can cause muscle tears and joint damage.

The science behind plyometrics

One of the principles of ply-sci is the **stretch shortening cycle** (SSC). This is made up of phases, where the muscles you're using are lengthened or stretched (the eccentric contraction) followed quickly by a shortening (the concentric contraction). The amortisation phase is the time in between the eccentric and concentric contractions. This is key, because how quickly you transition between the lengthening and shortening phase determines how effective the movement has been – essentially, the faster the better. If you take your sweet time getting from A to B, you'll lose any potential gains made between the contractions. It's the combination of these three phases that makes plyometrics such a powerful way to enhance the capacity of the muscles used.

There is a protective reflex in the body that can help prevent injury, and you can deliberately train and improve this reflex by doing plyometrics. When you are doing, or about to do, a movement that your brain thinks is dodgy (such as fall, slip or land badly), it will send a message to specific muscles to contract, basically as an act of damage control. Drawing on your central nervous system, plyometrics reinforces the brain–muscle connections (so, make friends with your CNS; think of it as the brains, while your muscles are the brawn). Think about when an older person has a fall – their leg might buckle, as their ankle will lack the mobility and strength to support them as they slip. Were they to do some plyometrics, they'd have trained their nervous system to adapt and support their day-to-day movements so that as soon as their foot was in the danger zone, their brain would start ringing the alarm bell and would send a signal to the muscles in the foot and ankle to straighten back up. This is the 'bouncing back' that you often hear about in reference to plyometrics, where it helps preserve muscle mass and muscle capability.

Speed and power

So, not only does SSC help prevent injury and correct imbalances, it also facilitates you to become better in whatever sport you do by improving speed and power. Just as it draws on the central nervous system to help prevent injury, it's this same mind–body connection that leads to greater training adaptions (this really comes into its own in the powerlifting section – see page 229).

Ground contact time (GCT): This is the amount of time your feet are in contact with the ground while doing the key moves. A **short cycle** is milliseconds on the floor, just like a sprinter would have (focus on their feet the next time you're watching a 100m race – it's mind-blowing how little time their feet spend on the ground; sprinters look more like they're flying than running). Obviously in disciplines like this, speed is everything – so you don't want to have your full foot on the floor, you want to do the minimum; quick as a flash and you're off again.

Plyometrics: let's do it

Plyometrics offers a variety of upper- and lower-body exercises which, as I've said, will improve strength, speed, power, reaction times, balance and coordination. If you've ever done HIIT or even some pre-workout warm-up drills, the chances are you've been doing some of these plyo movements already, without knowing. Lots of the movements are jump-based and challenge your muscles to work at a high capacity for short periods. It's the addition of these explosive jumps to your training regime that conditions the body to improve its strength and speed.

Look at how a basketball player moves with the ball, changes direction, pivoting quickly and following a lay-up with an explosive vertical jump off the ground for a slam-dunk. Or how a sprinter powers off the starting blocks with immense force. Plyometric training helps these athletes with their movements by improving control and coordination, conditioning muscles and tendons to make them more reactive.

Workouts

Lower-body plyometric training is almost always about using your body weight as resistance. You'll be thrusting, squatting, lunging and leaping like nobody's business. Upper-body workouts often involve using kit like a medicine ball (a weighted ball used in strength training to build muscles in the arm), which can be utilised in different ways, such as tossing the ball overhead and slamming it against the wall – a great way to release some pent-up aggression! Adding some plyo exercises to the start of your workout (rather than at the end, when your muscles are fatigued) will boost your strength and speed, and will really help your overall performance in whatever sport you're doing. If you'd like to see these and other exercises in action, go to my website (www.theomegaarmy.com/workout-videos).

Beginner's workout

Here's a handy little beginner's workout to get you started, devised by one of the *slowest* guys I know, Harry Aikines-Aryeetey (okay, maybe 'slow' isn't the *best* way to describe him . . .). Harry is an incredible Team GB sprinting champion, and plyometrics forms a fundamental part of his speed training. You don't need any special equipment and you can do it either at home or in a gym. See how you get on, but don't push yourself if it's your first time. If you're feeling any twinges in your joints, take a break.

EXERCISE	***TIME***	***SETS***	***REST BETWEEN EACH EXERCISE***
Ankle hops	30 seconds	4	10 seconds
Lateral hops	30 seconds	4	10 seconds
Squat jumps	30 seconds	4	10 seconds
180 jumps	30 seconds	4	10 seconds
Jump freezes	30 seconds	4	10 seconds
Jumps lunges	30 seconds	4	10 seconds
Tuck jumps	30 seconds	4	10 seconds

Elite workout

Cranking it up a notch, here's Harry's power-plyo session for a more advanced level. It's something an Olympic sprinter might incorporate into their training, so this should only be attempted if you have advanced experience of plyometrics. You'll need to work out your 1 rep max for this, i.e. the maximum you can do one repetition of an exercise for.

SS = super set (move quickly between the exercises without taking a break)

EXERCISE	***REPS***	***SETS***	***% OF 1 REP MAX***
Parallel squats	4	4 SS	70–80% (fast and reactive on the way up)
Box jumps/squat jumps	4	4	
Dumbbell or barbell Bulgarian split squats	4 on each leg	4 SS	80% (depending on space)
Bounds or jumping lunges	5	4	
Hip thrusts	5	4 SS	70–80% (depending on space)
Double foot jumps forward/standing broad jumps	3	4	

PLYOMETRICS

What plyometric training delivers: It conditions the body, improving overall athleticism. Enjoy noticing gains in any other training you do, too, where you'll be stronger and faster, and have more stamina and coordination.

Why it works: It builds muscle, particularly in the legs, making you stronger, more powerful, faster and more agile.

Physique: Toned, low body fat, strong lower body.

Pros: It's a good calorie-burner, so it can be a good option for those looking to lose weight. It improves overall strength, speed, endurance, co-ordination and agility, and it helps prevent injury, particularly in the joints.

Cons: Potential injury to ligaments, tendons, joints and muscles if exercises are done incorrectly, if you overdo it by not alternating exercises (e.g. if you do too many jumps, your knee joints can become damaged) or if you try to add a weightlifting element to the moves (which I've seen people try and it often doesn't end well).

Equipment: You can do an awful lot with body weight alone, but jump ropes, boxes, hurdles and medicine balls will mix up the range of exercises you can do.

Importance of technique: Learn how to land when squatting or box jumping.

PLAY

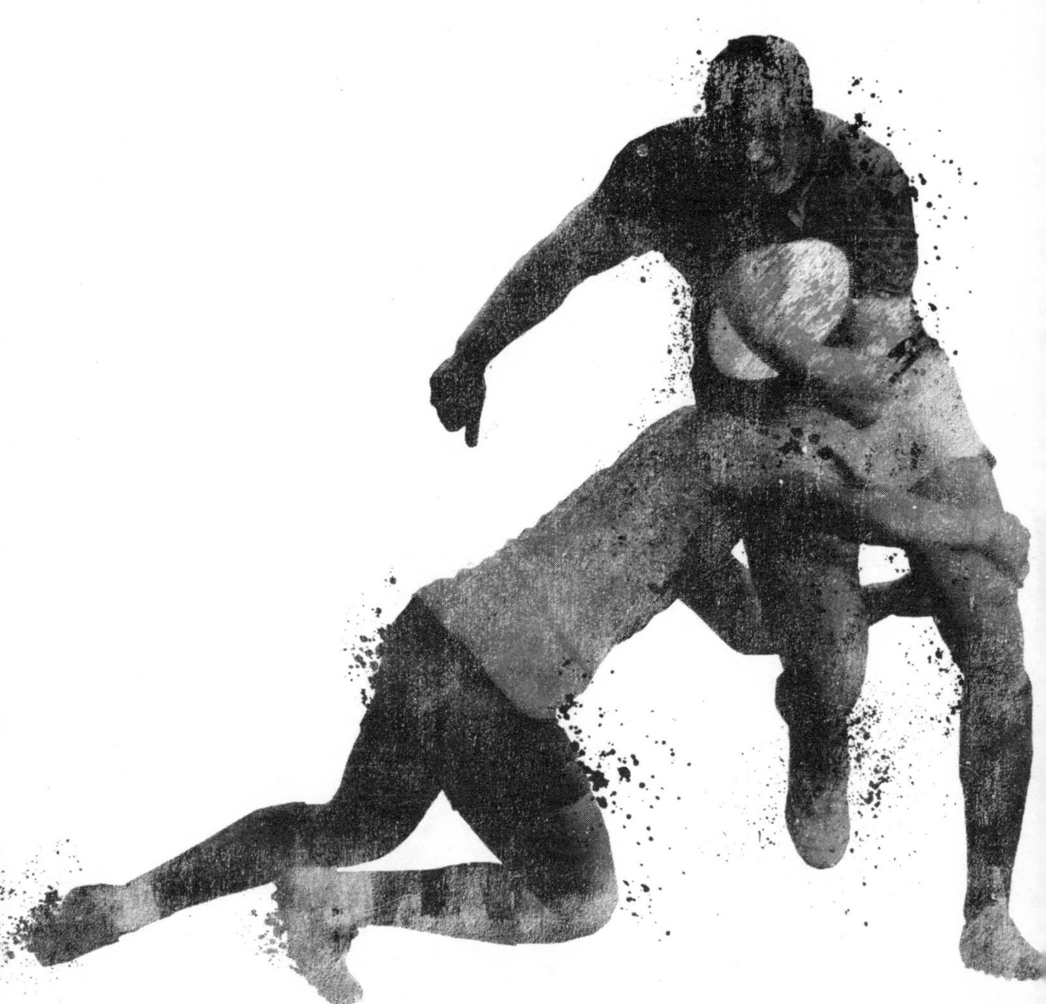

I'M NOW GOING to talk you through two team sports that are close to my heart – football and rugby, types of exercise that will advance your aerobic fitness, as well as your agility and stamina. But playing sports brings so many other benefits in addition to the physical ones. For one, sport is the ultimate equaliser, breaking down social barriers and bridging any perceived gaps between us.

Take football – a universal language. When I'm on the set of an ad campaign for Nike, Puma, Adidas or whoever, working as a sports choreographer, often the first thing I do to help everyone feel relaxed is get out a football. A simple kickabout immediately breaks the ice – pretensions or hierarchy go out the window as everyone gets involved, from the athlete at the centre of the ad to the camera man, the runner and the extras. After a few minutes of two-touch (a game where everyone stands in a circle and the aim is to pass the ball round, keeping it up in the air with only two touches, one to control and one to pass it to someone else), there's no star anymore and everyone feels that bit more chilled. And whoever messes up by letting the ball fall to the floor will get an ear flicking, whether it's the make-up artist or Cesc Fàbregas – no ear is safe. Anyway, high jinks like these relax people and can be especially helpful when dealing with anyone who is more reserved. It can also defuse any ructions that might be brewing. If you're bantering and joking in good company, stress levels will plummet. Isn't laughter the antidote to stress? Laugh at yourself, laugh with others, and you can't go far wrong.

There are football and rugby clubs everywhere, but if you're looking for something more informal or ad hoc, just grab your mates for a kickabout or throw-about in the park – you'll be building your fitness, getting a bit of fresh air and letting off some steam while you're at it.

FOOTBALL

> 'Never lose sight of yourself. It doesn't matter what others are doing; focus on what you want to achieve and you'll get a better performance.'
>
> GEMMA DAVISON, ENGLAND AND TOTTENHAM HOTSPUR FOOTBALLER

Football was everything to me when I was a kid. It was the common language of the lads where I lived, and there was often a knock at the door from another boy, football under the arm, asking my old pair if I could come out to the green and play. Jumpers thrown down as goalposts, endless energy, good banter with some occasional ructions, and always returning home from dinner in a muddy school uniform.

One of my earliest memories of football was watching Ireland play against Italy on telly in the 1994 World Cup in America. When the players strode out onto the pitch before kick-off, the Irish fans in the stadium started singing the national anthem (which, hilariously, a lot of the players didn't know, having not actually grown up in Ireland and only being connected to the country by a parent or grand-parent – a bit tenuous some might say!). Anyway, I was belting it out at home to the screen, watching some of my heroes file out. I felt a bit of a connection to one of them, Paul McGrath – I'm convinced my parents named me after him; I was born the year after he was capped for Ireland. He was a role model to me and everyone at school would call me by that name (what with both of us being Paul and Black you can imagine I was pretty popular after the match!). If you ask any Irish person old enough to remember, they'll be able to recount this particular game with the accuracy of it happening yesterday (and with a tear in their eye): Ray Houghton's infamous winning goal against Italy, giving Ireland a great boost in the World Cup. (I'm not crying – you're crying!) Everything changed after this. I'd always loved football, but I was a boy possessed after such a victory. Football took over most of my waking thoughts (I was only around eight, so didn't have many other pressing matters to deal with). I remember thinking that if Paul McGrath was willing to die for the Irish jersey, then I was too. Okay, they were knocked out in the next round, but come on . . . Ireland beating Italy – that was incredible!

When I was around ten I started playing for a team called Verona (sounds glamorous but was actually just the local side where I lived in Dublin). After a few years, when I was a teenager, I got a trial for Shamrock Rovers, a top-league youth division team in Dublin, and played with them for two seasons. I was training about three or four times a week, so this is when I really started living and breathing football, and wondered if maybe I could make a career out of it. I then started playing for St Patrick's Athletic, another top team, where I built up a bit of a rep when scouts came to see games, watching out for new talent.

Aged nineteen, I moved to London to play professionally, and it was here that I trained under first-class coaches. When I stopped playing football professionally, I studied to be a football coach myself. I had been lucky enough to have observed some incredible coaches, and two in particular really influenced me: Russell Wilcox at Scunthorpe and Rob Garvey at Dagenham & Redbridge both had amazing energy; they had an aura about them that inspired me. When I did my coaching and PT training, it was them I often thought about. Their knowledge, as well as their zeal for life, really stayed with me. I wanted to be able to inspire people to love sport and fitness in the same way that they had motivated me on the pitch.

I've talked already about when I was first trying to make it into professional football. I thought I was raring to go in terms of fitness, until, that was, I actually tried to play a game. Off the pitch, I was fit enough to keep running all day if I wanted to, which lulled me into a false sense of security thinking I was in tip-top condition. Fifteen minutes into my first game, though, and I was a mess. Where I had been used to running at a consistent pace over long stretches, my energy systems weren't sufficiently trained for a change of pace that would need to include stopping and starting, and sprinting. I couldn't do it, because even though I had good overall aerobic fitness, I wasn't match-fit and I couldn't keep up. That's why footballers do pre-season games rather than just jogging training.

There have been strides made in recent years to bring more women into football (about time). Twenty million UK viewers tuned in to see the incredible performance of England's women's team in 2019's World Cup, and I was one of them, sitting on the edge of my seat watching the semi-final against the US. While I wish there had been an Irish women's team to support, England is my other home and it would have been nice to see them win. And here's hoping for an Irish team (male or female) in the next World Cup – I'll light a candle!

Team spirit

The benefits to your physical health that football bring are clear, and the mental ones are very much up there too. You'll be hard-pushed to find an area the world over that doesn't have a local team, even if it's an informal once-a-week park kickabout. Its ubiquity is one of the brilliant things about football, and even if you're not the best ever player, you can have a fantastic time being part of a team. It can give you such a lift, it can make the actual exercise you do almost peripheral.

Training workout

Here's a simple strength routine that will help to build the muscles in your legs, and improve balance and coordination, which you can do two or three times a week. Strong leg muscles can help keep good alignment in the whole body, which in turn helps to prevent injuries such as knee issues. You can do this on the pitch in a training session or even at home while you watch TV. If you're unsure of how to do any of these warm-up exercises, go to www.theomegaarmy.com/workout-videos, where I'll take you through them.

Warm-up

EXERCISE	***REPS***	***SETS***	***REST***
Lunge walks	15 on both sides	3	30 seconds
Lateral walks	15 on both sides	3	30 seconds
Jump squats	15	3	30 seconds
Glute bridge	30 seconds	3	30 seconds
Single leg deadlift	15 on both sides	3	30 seconds
Standing calf raise	15	3	30 seconds
Side plank	30 seconds on each side	3	30 seconds

Running

To play football at a decent level, you need to be able to keep up with the ball. Over the course of a match, you could be running some 10k, meaning stamina is essential. On top of that, you need to be able to stop and start quickly, so you'll need to train in a way that develops your different energy systems. I want to refer you back to Fartlek training on page 125, where you will be alternating weekly runs between sprinting short distances, sometimes slow-jogging and going at a medium pace for longer runs. It's a tried and tested way to build speed and endurance, preventing the body from plateauing.

Drills

There's no fixed amount of time you need to do this for; depending on your training session on the day or how much time you have, it could be anything from a few minutes to 20–30 minutes.

Keep ball: This is a great drill to start a training session, for getting everyone in the mood before a match or even a kickabout with your friends in the park. With everyone standing in a circle, the aim is to keep passing the ball while not letting it drop to the ground.

Speed work: Lay out cones and practise dribbling the ball around them as quickly as possible while maintaining control. Play around with the spacing of the cones to make it more challenging.

Technique and control: Very simply, you might practise skills like heading the ball, so get into pairs with one person kicking or throwing the ball up and the other heading it back.

Five-a-side: The end of the session should always finish with some actual football! Depending on how many you are, get into small teams, preferably four, five or six people a side, and play! If you're playing in a competitive league, this is your time to shine, where you show the coaches your 'tekkers' so that they pick you for the match at the weekend.

FOOTBALL

What football delivers: Great aerobic fitness, team bonding and the pleasure of being outdoors.

Why it works: It involves a lot of running as well as agility drills that improve skill and overall performance.

Physique: Lean, low body fat and strong legs.

Pros: You'll develop endurance as well as adapting to short bursts of energy. If you join a team, you'll enjoy the social element, endorphins and being outdoors.

Cons: Like most sports, injuries can happen while playing football, but that shouldn't put you off, especially when playing at an amateur level.

Equipment: Football boots (if playing on grass), trainers and a ball.

Importance of technique: Skills drills will help you finesse techniques, and when you're playing under a coach you will work on practices specific to your position on the pitch. But even if you're playing more informally, say with friends in the park, you will notice improvements with every game.

RUGBY

> 'The values rugby teaches you can be used in every walk of life – like shaking hands with someone you've just been to war with.'
>
> JOHNNY SEXTON, RUGBY CAPTAIN OF IRELAND AND WORLD RUGBY PLAYER OF THE YEAR 2018

After many years of being married to football, my mistress rugby came knocking. I had always played at school, but it'd come second fiddle to football. Once I got properly into it again, however, it was love. My older brother Martin was an amazing player (or 'egg-chaser', as rugby players are known!). He was the lord of school rugby. I still remember him running past six players any time he got the ball; he was like a cheetah. He then went on to play with the prestigious Leinster under-21s in Ireland before moving to the UK to play for Plymouth Albion. He inspired me to get back into rugby. I was in my late twenties and still pretty fast still off the back of the recent football training combined with spending a good bit of time at the gym. So I decided to give it a whirl.

Nigeria had a 7s team and I joined them. It was pretty cool that the first bit of rugby I played since school was international, and for the country where my old pair were born. I was obviously a lot less experienced than the rest of the team, but I was considered fast and fairly fearless, so they'd pass me the ball and I'd run! The Nigerian 7s trained in Surrey, not far from Esher Rugby Club, and I got in touch with their coach to see if I could play with them. I ended up doing that for four years. I was full-time at the start, but then dropped down to being semi-pro. I was playing pretty regularly over the next three seasons and I also got to play for Harlequin's A-league squad, which scratched an itch, as my friend Matt Garvey, who played for Bath, had once told me I'd never make it in rugby, having spent so much time previously playing football. But there I was on the same field as Maro Itoje, playing against Saracens. It was quite an honour to be on the same pitch as Itoje (he's lucky I got injured or I'd probably be running over him every Saturday . . .). It was a brilliant time in my life and the values I learned there shaped the person I am now.

Rugby culture

If you've never considered playing rugby, I'd urge you to do so. You can dip your toe in at whatever level, even if it's just playing tag rugby once a week with friends in the park.

Rugby is an incredible sport for building strength, agility and endurance, but also for teaching determination and problem-solving, which is why I think it's great for kids too. There are two strands of this sport, rugby league and rugby union, but here I'm going to be concentrating on rugby league only.

There are thirteen players – forwards, who do the heavy grunt work, and those at the back, who do all the speed work, in addition to a scrum half, who connect the forwards to the backs. If you've played any rugby or watched a game, you'll know it's a very physical sport that has many high-contact elements – scrums, rucks, tackling. You can tackle a player who's carrying the ball anywhere on the body apart from the head, neck and, in a more recent (and, in my opinion, softie) rule, the shoulders. So, on the one hand it might seem to the untrained eye as kind of brutish and wild, but in reality it's a game of rules and manners. And yes, some of the rules are kind of eccentric, but when you play, you have faith in them and come to understand that they're there for the greater good and for the beauty of the game.

Players respect the rules, too; what the ref says goes. So, whereas you might see a football player pleading with a ref to change a decision, getting all up in their grill and sometimes becoming aggro, that doesn't happen in rugby, where only the captain communicates with the ref. That was a learning curve for me when I moved from football to rugby – I used to swear blue murder at football refs when a ruling didn't go my way, and when I called out the ref's decision during my first rugby match (thug that I was!), it was my own team mates I got a bollocking from. It's just not the done thing in rugby, because respect is a fundamental tenet of the game. Yes, there's the odd swing thrown (guilty!) at the opposition, but at the end of the game, every opponent's hand is shaken and a tunnel is formed by one team to applaud and cheer the other side and vice versa. The referee also walks through the tunnel, so even if you thought they'd been unfair during the game, you get over it by clapping them through. Research carried out on sport has actually suggested that touch and affection improves the outcomes of games, and I really see that being the case in rugby. It's a beautiful thing that brings respect to life and it's something I wish football would learn from. The same goes for the fans; whereas in football, you need to separate the away and home side watching matches, at rugby they're all mixed together and there's never any trouble.

The camaraderie in rugby is second-to-none, and if you

join a rugby club, you'll get as many social benefits as you will physical ones. It's like joining a family. When it comes to finding a tribe, I'd pick rugby over any other sport. The ethos is that no person is left behind; your team will spur you on and look after you, always willing you to do well.

So, if you're wanting to make some new friends, look in your local area (there are men's and women's clubs all over the place) to see if there's a club, or you could also ask around to see if anyone wants to start a tag rugby team.

Rugby training

Rugby is about conditioning the whole body so that it is prepared for what will be thrown at it during a match. If you join a team, a training session might look a little like the one outlined below. Otherwise, this is a plan you can easily follow at home or in the park. Ideally you'd be doing this with a couple of friends, as the drills rely on passing the ball to someone. Obviously it'll differ from training with a club (unless you happen to own a scrum machine in your back garden), where forwards and backs work to develop skills specific to their roles on the pitch, for example practising lineouts, as well as working on any team strategies the coach may be devising.

So, this is a more general workout that will support your body if you're thinking about playing rugby or even, as I mentioned a bit earlier, if you play informally with friends, where you throw the ball about for fun. These exercises are good for building leg strength and improving agility. The skills blocks are good fun and would also be great activities if you ever find yourself needing to entertain kids in a park or garden.

Workout

Warm-ups

In a good rugby session, the warm-up is pretty comprehensive rather than a short, token stretch or quick jog on the spot, and it will include a strength and conditioning element. If you don't spend time firing up key muscle groups in your shoulders, back, core and legs before your session, it can increase stiffness afterwards as well as putting you at higher risk of injury.

Banded glute activation: Place resistance bands around your feet and knees and get into a quarter squat position. Walk to the left for 20 steps and then do 20 steps to the right; then go forwards for 20 steps and backwards for 20 steps. You glutes should be feeling the burn!

Banded bridges: Lie on the ground on your back, with the soles of your trainers on the ground and your feet and knees hip-width apart. Place a resistance band just above your knees and lift your back up off the ground, squeezing your glutes as you go. Repeat for 30 seconds to 1 minute.

Lying hamstring extension: Lying flat on your back, have one leg flat out on the ground and the other stretched up towards the sky. Hold the back of the shin (or further up the leg around the thigh if you can't reach lower down) and bring the leg in towards your body. Hold the stretch for about 30 seconds before swapping legs.

Shoulder loosen (this is only an option if you're training with someone): With a buddy, tap your right shoulder against their right shoulder. It should be firm but it shouldn't hurt. Alternate between right and left for about 30 seconds.

Chainsaw shoulder opener: Get down on all fours and, keeping your left palm on the ground and the left arm straight, stretch your right arm under your left one. Now pull your right arm as if you're starting up a chainsaw, repeating for about 30 seconds before switching sides.

Skills block

These are drills used to practise and finesse ball skills, but they'll also boost fitness.

Conditioning drill: If you're in a park (rather than on a pitch, where these markings will already be in place), use cones (or jumpers if you don't have any!) to roughly mark out 5m, 10m and 15m lines. At a good pace (not quite a sprint), start at the 10m line. Run to the 15m line and lie down on the ground before hopping back up and running to the 5m line. Keep alternating the lines you run to and remember each time to lie down on the ground and spring up again.

Passing drill: There are many different passing drills out there, but a very simple one to start with is to form a line (however many of you there are; this will work even with two people, though) and as you're running, pass the ball sideways down the line, and back up again. Short and long passing drills are a part of all rugby training, so vary the distances between you when passing the ball.

Cone drills and ladder drills: As with football, place cones and/or a fitness ladder down on the ground and use them as markers for running though, practising quick footwork to improve agility.

Cool-down

If you're at the park or on the pitch, do a lap at a slow-to-moderate jog before stretching out your calves, hamstrings, quads, chest, triceps and shoulders. All told, it should take around 10–15 minutes.

Hamstrings: Begin by standing upright, feet together and firmly planted on the floor. Bend over, reaching your hands down to touch your toes.

Calves: Standing straight up, put your weight onto your right foot, lifting your heel and coming onto the balls of your feet or tippy toes. Release down slowly and repeat on the other side.

Quads: With one foot planted firmly on the ground, bend the other knee and kick your foot back towards your backside, using your hand to hold it here. After you feel a good stretch, repeat on the other side.

Back and shoulders: Come down onto your knees in front of a bench or a chair (as if you were about to pray). Place your elbows on the bench, with your arms reaching up towards the ceiling, palms together. Your eyes should be looking down at the floor, keeping the spine and the neck aligned (rather than your neck and head bending towards the floor). Hang out here for as long as is comfortable.

Shoulders: Get down on all fours. Stretch your right arm under your left one, resting your right shoulder on the ground. Hang out here for about 30 seconds and then switch to the other side.

Triceps: Standing straight with feet hip-width apart, stretch the right arm up to the ceiling, bend the elbow and reach the right hand down between your shoulder blades.

Place the left hand on the right elbow, gently pressing the elbow down. Repeat on the other side.

RUGBY

What rugby delivers: Strength, power, endurance and agility.

Why it works: It builds upper- and lower-body strength as well as aerobic fitness.

Physique: Depending on your position, you're likely to be muscly. Rugby players are often big but able to run.

Pros: The loving atmosphere of a team who become your family, as well as fitness that draws on different energy systems.

Cons: It's a high-impact sport and if you are playing matches you may be injured.

Equipment: Shirt, shorts, studded boots and a gumshield. Some players wear scrum hats and some tape their legs, which helps them to get a grip in a lineout.

Importance of technique: Rugby is a game of skill and strategy, which is why practising techniques forms a big part of the training (in addition to building fitness).

STRETCH

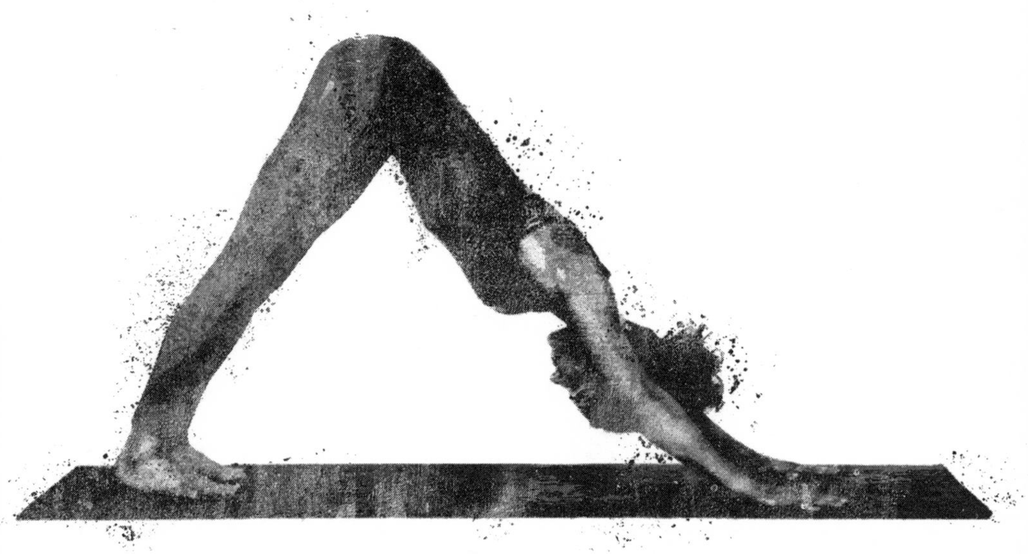

THIS SECTION IS all about taking care of your body by stretching, strengthening and mobilising in order to help prevent injury, and keeping it supple and resilient so that it can support you in everyday tasks and in any other training you do.

Incorporating yoga and mobility exercises into my regime is relatively new to me and I don't want to be a stretching bore (there are enough of those on the 'Gram as it is), but it has been a game-changer for me (particularly the yin yoga I do). I'll explain this more in the mobility section coming up, but essentially I always overlooked stretching, never giving it the time of day. Failing to do proper warm-ups caused me a lot of pain (though, at the time, I didn't know that a bit of yoga could have resolved so much of it) and impacted my weightlifting progress. Honestly, I never got into it or gave it much thought because I was too focused on lifting, lifting, lifting. I didn't register that increased flexibility or balance between the left and right side of my body would make me a more competent powerlifter.

There are many ways to help maintain your body. Here I talk about yoga, general mobility work, gymnastics and calisthenics, but there are so many others out there to explore if you're curious, such as Pilates or Eastern practices like quigong. Many are low-impact routes to whole-body health as they combine elements of movement and breathing, with some also incorporating mindfulness and meditation.

YOGA

> 'Yoga is a time to get out of your head and into your heart. It's vital for our wellbeing that we take time to slow down our minds and connect with our breath. Postures are the best way to release tension – the feeling you get at the end of a session when your mind is clear and you've untied the knots in your body is so peaceful.'
>
> PARIS PARLE, YOGA EXPERT

Here's a little quiz to start you off in this section. Answers to the below on a postcard:

- What will help tone your body, build muscle and improve strength?
- What will make you more flexible and coordinated, and aid your balance?
- What can help fix back pain and even prevent arthritis, osteoarthritis and general aches?
- What can do you if you're feeling worried or frazzled?
- What will lower your blood pressure, improve concentration and help you focus better on work or your home life?
- What exercise can you try if you're unfit and inflexible?
- What can bring you spiritual enlightenment?

Look no further: the answer to all of these questions is (yes, you guessed it): yoga!

Okay, you might have seen that coming. Really, though, out of all the exercises I suggest in this book, you might be surprised to hear that this is the one I'd really urge you to try. Sore back? Yoga. Stiff joints? Yoga? Bad mood? Yoga. It's the answer to almost everything.

Yoga has seen a massive rise in popularity in the West over the past decade but, of course, it's an ancient practice that began in India. Until relatively recently, yoga would have been seen in this country as being a bit 'out there', something a bit hippie or New Age, but thankfully it's mainstream these days. For many, yoga is a whole lifestyle, almost like a religion or a state of mind, which ties into how they live in the world. The spiritual side appeals to a lot of people, but you can always sack off the candles and chanting if you find all that a bit 'no-ta-not-for-me'. Some people are put off by yoga, but really you can think of it as just stretching. Every pro athlete and sportsperson does it, even if they call it something else. Don't let any preconceptions or fears – about being too stiff/too old/too unfit to begin yoga – get in your way.

The benefits of yoga are well established, and you'd be as likely now to hear your GP prescribing you a spot of yoga as you would a faith healer. Some of the health benefits are listed in the quiz above; yoga will not only contribute to your overall maintenance, reduce joint pain and make you stronger, it can also prevent certain conditions. A common reason why people turn to it is, like Pilates, to strengthen the core. This in turn can help with back pain. The spine is a focus-point in yoga – it's all about protecting it, strengthening it and keeping it stable. In developed countries, lots of us tend to spend long hours either hunched over a desk, driving or generally sitting down too much, which means that the number of people suffering with bad backs is on the rise. Doing some yoga every day can be the best cure.

The psychological benefits have just as many bragging

rights. Many people find it a stress-buster, calming anxious thoughts, compulsive behaviour and making them feel more positive generally. It can help slow the pace of life down (we all need that – surely it was never meant to be this fast?), quietening the mind, and when you're feeling a bit more peaceful, you might tap into your self-reliance and inner confidence. Many people find this particularly effective when combined with meditation, and many classes do include a silent or guided meditation. Also, as a result of feeling more relaxed and less stressed, many people find their sleep improves.

User-friendly

The beauty of yoga is that there's a practice out there for you that will match your needs on the day (I list some of the popular ones on page 170). This flexibility works particularly well if you ever decide to do online sessions (either free ones or those that are more like virtual classes, happening live, where your instructor can see you and give guidance). In the first instance (at the very least), though, I would recommend going to an in-person class so that the instructor can observe your movements and give feedback on them, correcting postures where necessary. Many yoga-lovers attend regular classes or they follow their own practice at home, and lots of people do a bit of both.

A practice session can vary anywhere from a few minutes to around an hour and a half. If you're feeling a bit apprehensive about going to a class for the first time, get a friend to tag along. Some studios and gyms will even allow you to observe a class before doing one for real. Some classes include meditation or breathing exercises, while others are shorter and more exercise-focused, so just do what feels right. If you do attend a class but don't get what all the fuss is about, try another one – like any fitness regime, there are brilliant teachers out there and also less good ones. Your instructor can make a huge difference to your experience of yoga, so if you're not vibing off yours, choose another one before giving up. Similarly, try different types of yoga to find the one that suits your temperament or goals best.

Yoga is not about competition (and this is something I frequently need to remind myself, as I'm always trying to win, or at the very least beat my own record). That is very much not the ethos. It's not about perfecting your technique or showing off how stretchy you are, but focusing on little improvements that make you feel good. So for this one, get rid of the push-yourself-until-you-puke-into-a-bucket mentality!

Any age

You are never too old to start yoga and to reap the benefits. The beauty of yoga is that you follow your body, only going as far with a position as is comfortable. If any of them are prohibitive, no worries, just move on to the next. Yoga isn't all headstands and one-arm crow pose; there are many positions that are done sitting or lying down. As yoga is a form of resistance training (using body weight as resistance), it's beneficial to older adults as it can improve bone strength (in some cases helping to prevent conditions like osteoporosis), boost overall fitness and lower blood pressure. It's also a good option for pregnant women who want to stay active through low-impact exercise; there are many classes designed for pregnancy, with movements that can be adapted around bumps. Some teachers of pregnancy yoga will also lead mums through exercises that may help encourage the baby into optimal in-utero positions for birth (useful during the final few weeks of gestation). There are even postures that some mums use during labour, which some say ease pain and encourage calm.

While we're on the subject of age, you're also never too *young* to start. So by all means get your kids involved – you'll be setting a great example if they see you practising and they'll love joining in, if only to show you how much more flexible they are! Little 'uns are naturally bendy, and some schools who have added yoga to their physical education curriculum report that children have a better attention span in lessons.

Postures

Knows as *asanas* in the biz, there are hundreds of these, and the more broad your practice the more postures you will incorporate. You'll probably find that there are some classic poses you keep coming back to, or others that feel great, which you deliberately try to incorporate if you are freestyling rather than following a class. For example, a sun salutation is a sequence of poses, variations of which include positions such as downward dog and child's pose, often repeated as a warm-up at the beginning of a session. Again, there are a lot of variations and no one 'right' way. A sun salutation can be a super transferable warm-up for other sports you're playing too, so feel free to take it out on the open road, doing a few salutations before another training session.

When you start doing yoga, you'll gradually get to know the positions through repetition. I would recommend getting comfortable with as many as you can under the guidance of a teacher if possible, before going it alone at home. That's because your alignment in a posture can be affected if a part of your stance is even a little bit off – for example, if the angle of your foot isn't quite right, it will have a knock-on effect on your knees, hips and upper body. You might not be able to tell unless an experienced instructor is observing you, who will then gently correct you – sometimes it's a matter of moving a centimetre that makes a big difference.

Some classes like to focus on a specific area of the body at a time, and this can be really effective if you have some niggles you want to target or a part of the body that you want to strengthen, for example. So, one session might include lots of hip postures, another might be focused on back exercises to strengthen the spine, while others might target the whole body.

Most classes end in a pose called *shavasana* (corpse pose), where you get to lie down and doze off if you like. Mood.

Yoga and the breath

Yoga and deep breathing are the best of buddies. *Pranayama* is the practice of conscious, controlled breathing that you can (and should) extend way beyond the yoga studio and incorporate into everyday life. If you've ever heard the advice to take long, deep breaths, especially when you're stressed, it's not just to distract yourself from your unease. It's because it immediately relaxes your parasympathetic nervous system and slows down your heart rate. If you've ever noticed yourself holding your breath, or taking shallow, shorter breaths, when you're feeling scared, annoyed or anxious, then try breathing in through your nose for four counts and exhaling out through your mouth for six counts – repeat this four times and your nervous system will high-five you from the inside out.

There are many breathing exercises out there to discover.

When you start out with yoga (and I would definitely still consider myself a beginner), it might take a while to coordinate your breathing with the postures, but gradually it becomes more intuitive and after a while you won't need reminding by the teacher to inhale or exhale at particular stages. I have found that this focusing on the breath also helps when I'm weightlifting, as breathing dynamics also play a part there (on page 238 I give instructions for directing the breath through the abdomen, which helps protect the back while doing certain exercises like weightlifting).

Which practice to choose?

There are so many different types of yoga, you could spend years practising and not explore all the variations. Some are more dynamic and will have you working up a sweat, while others have you doing just a few poses but holding them for longer. The environment can also change with yoga – typically classes happen in a studio, but they can also be done out in the open air, by candlelight; some even take place in silence, with the instructor teaching through movement rather than by voice.

There are specific classes that will guide you through postures for particular aches and pains or areas you want to work on in the body, so you'll see some advertised as 'yoga for upper-body strength' or 'yoga for back pain'. There are also athlete-specific ones so, for example, if you do boxing training, there are classes for boxers in mind where the key muscles used in the ring will be focused on in a yogic way. Other classes are themed by a feeling they're trying to target, e.g. 'yoga to help you sleep' or 'yoga to boost energy'. And then many don't advertise a specific promise and are instead just labelled by the type of yoga they are. I'm listing here some of the fairly common strands, where you should have no trouble finding a class or an online session. Some people find a type of yoga they fall in love with, while others might alternate between different practices. Sometimes instructors will incorporate poses from different ones within the same lesson. I've thrown a few wildcards in there too, just in case you want to diversify. Without a doubt, you'll find one that appeals – even if it's just you in your PJs in your living room.

Yin yoga

This type of yoga is focused on the muscles, tendons, ligaments and joints, which is why I find it so helpful, because by improving my range of motion it supports my powerbuilding. It's restorative, too, because it releases tension and any physical discomfort I might be in from lifting weights.

Hatha yoga

This is a great place to start, as it tends to be quite gentle and slower-paced than some of the other types of yoga. Classes are often structured around a flow of postures, with each *asana* paving the way for the next in the sequence. It usually includes a meditation or breathing exercises and is good for all levels of experience.

Ashtanga yoga

This tends to be a bit pacier than Hatha, as you flow through a set of dynamic sequences. While challenging, however, it can still be enjoyed by all levels. The postures are done with fairly swift transitions, but you can always go at your own speed. Remember, it's not a competition and no teacher will flog you for slowing down.

Iyengar yoga

B. K. S. Iyengar was an Indian yogi who was among the first to teach Westerners the delights of stretchiness. This strand is widely practised and it can be a good place for beginners because it's not super-fast and it focuses on being precise, meaning you'll get a good grasp of the positions.

Bikram yoga

This type of yoga's main claim to fame is that it is done in a room heated to around 35–40°C, with a high humidity level. For this reason it's not everyone's idea of a picnic, and it's not suitable for pregnant women or those with a heart condition, among others. The addition of heat is intended to boost flexibility. Spoiler alert: there are twenty-six postures in Bikram yoga and you follow the same sequence in every class.

Floating yoga

Sometimes called aerial yoga, this is where harnesses and slings are used for an antigravity workout. To call it yoga might be a bit of a stretch (sorry, couldn't help myself); I'm not sure it would meet with the approval of a hardcore yogi. Let's just say it's inspired by some of the positions in yoga that you do while suspended, the idea being you can stretch more deeply without having your body weight to support.

Laughter yoga

I was delighted when I recently heard about this, as I've always been a fan of using laughter to lighten the load. This variation started out in Mumbai, where a doctor came up with this yoga spin-off in an attempt to use laughter as a form of therapy. It involves stretching, clapping, breathing exercises and some japes to get you howling. This is best done in a real-life, in-person class, as in relies on a group bursting into spontaneous LOLs (it's contagious as we all know). Fifteen minutes or more of laughter (whether it's genuine or fake) triggers a dose of happy hormones. On top of that, having a good old belly laugh is a type of aerobic exercise, so it stimulates blood flow around the body and has a similar effect on the stomach as sit-ups. Does it work in making people happier and more relaxed in the long term? God knows. But I reckon it's worth a go.

Dog yoga

Get your hound to join you for a spot of downward dog (ahem . . .). Don't have a dog? No problem – take your goat instead. Pet yoga has a dedicated fanbase, with peeps bringing their furry friends to a class (often held in parks) to stretch alongside them. Some people even lift up their small dogs for the standing poses (better suited for a pug than Great Dane). Mad as a box of frogs? I think so. But whatever floats your boat!

Nude yoga

Say no more – I'm there. *Namaste.*

Postures and sequences

There are any number of combinations of postures you can put together, and once you find your groove you can develop your own, putting together a series of movements depending on your intention or goal for the session. Here's a simple stretch-sequence I sometimes do when I get up in the morning (provided I don't have a toddler throwing a Sylvanian in my face). It's useful if you're feeling stiff, particularly in the back, either from a bad night's sleep or from working out. You can do it at any time of day, and it usually takes me about five minutes, but there are no timings or number of repetitions to follow, unlike a lot of my other workouts, and that's because you should just do what feels good. You can make this as calm or as dynamic as you fancy.

1. Begin on all fours flowing through **cat** and **cow** poses. With knees under your hips, lift up your chest and face towards the ceiling (this is the cow part), drawing your shoulders back. From here, move your face down to look at the floor between your hands and bring a gentle curve to your spine (a little like a cat), rounding your upper back towards the ceiling. Flow gently between the poses.
2. From there go into **downward dog**, by lifting up from all fours with your hands firmly planted on the floor, stretching your backside up towards the ceiling, straightening your legs and aiming your heels towards the floor (don't worry if they don't reach it). Now 'walk the dog' by lifting your heels up and down, as if walking on the spot.

3. Walk your feet up to the top of the mat and do some **standing roll-downs**, leading from your head and gradually rolling your upper body down through each vertebra with your fingers stretched out towards the mat.
4. Come back into **downward dog** for a hang-out.
5. Gently come down to the floor, lying on your back, and come into **reclined pigeon pose** by bending your knees and placing both feet on the floor quite close to your backside. Lift one shin in towards you and place your lower leg or ankle on top of the other thigh. Hold this position or gradually increase the stretch by nudging the thigh towards your upper body. You can also lift your shoulders up off the floor to increase the intensity of the stretch – but only if this feels comfortable. Swap legs and do each side for roughly the same amount of time.
6. Lying on your back, sinking your lower back into the floor, do a **knees-to-chest** pose. Give your knees a hug and have a little rock from side to side.
7. Finish in **child's pose** – get onto all fours and stretch your bum back towards your feet, relaxing down towards them. You can keep your arms stretched outwards with palms firmly on the floor or resting down alongside your body.

When you're getting started, don't worry about getting these postures 'perfect' (whatever that means); as you practise, you will naturally progress. (You should see me doing some of them where I'm more like a buffalo than a graceful gazelle . . .)

YOGA

What yoga delivers: whole-body conditioning and stress release.

Why it works: It encourages good alignment and builds strength using body-weight as resistance.

Physique: This will vary depending on how much you practise but it helps build muscle and keeps the body limber.

Pros: Mental clarity and calm, physical strength, improved posture, flexibility, co-ordination and balance.

Cons: Very few, if any! Yoga is one of the safest low-impact exercises you can do. Try to ensure you are positioning yourself correctly (going to a class, particularly when you're starting out, will help with this) to avoid damaging joints such as the knees.

Equipment: Yoga mat, brick, block and straps can be helpful, but if you don't have those, a blanket or towel, a cushion and a belt make good substitutes.

Importance of technique: Optimal positioning is important to get the most from your practice and to avoid injury, which is why I suggest attending a class (or classes) if you're a beginner. Proper alignment will help you get stronger and more flexible, enabling you to hold positions for longer and progress to more advanced postures.

MOBILITY

I could also call this section 'yoga or Pilates for sceptics', because that's what it is – stretching without the incense and gong bathing. The word 'yoga' seems to scare the bejesus out of some people, particularly the men I know. Probably because they're worried about letting rip in a busy class while in downward dog. I mean, haven't we've all done it? I'll confess if you do.

Until fairly recently, I used to hurt just walking around. I was so stiff from my gym work, even the simplest day-to-day tasks gave me grief. Lifting weights does put a serious toll on the body. For over a decade I was shelling out eye-watering amounts to chiropractors in an attempt to sort out my creaking bones, which would feel so much better after they'd worked a bit of magic, only the pain would creep back within days, meaning I was often returning weekly for the pleasure of them conducting what felt like a karate chop down my spine. They provided short-term relief but, in my experience, didn't address the root cause of the pain.

Tired of feeling like a ninety-year-old, I booked a session with an osteopath, and it brought about a lightbulb moment. Yes, he could see I was clearly suffering from lower-back and shoulder pain, but he identified where this was stemming from and gave me exercises to do at home. I was blown away by how much these improved the discomfort I'd been in for so many years. He then had a look at why my knees often felt like they'd been rolled through a mangle and worked out that it was all to do with how my feet were positioned during squats. So all this time I'd thought my knees were the problem, and it was actually just because I wasn't spreading my toes out and gripping the floor effectively during a squat, which had a knock-on effect on my ankles and meant I was loading too much on my knees. If you've ever done Pilates or yoga, where there is often emphasis on planting your feet firmly on the ground, rooting you down, then you'll be ahead of the game.

I tried my newfound love of mobility exercises out on my mumsy, who'd been in daily agony for as long as I could remember, and had been spending my inheritance on her regular appointments with the chiropractor, with no long-term improvement. I got her to start doing a few very simple stretches each morning, and it has transformed her overall mobility and massively improved her lower-back pain. She can even walk a half marathon now, so for her these mobility exercises have been truly life-changing.

Obviously, the benefits of not being in pain are a no-brainer – people who suffer from chronic pain are often, unsurprisingly, worn down physically and mentally, because it takes such a toll. But increased mobility will also make your training much more effective, so I do mobility exercises before each session to prime my body, and I also do them every morning as a part of my wake-up-and-move routine. They are a form of self-massage and deep stretching that loosens the muscles and helps relieve tightness. They lead your muscles, tendons and joints through a full range of motion, which will maximise whatever training you do afterwards. For example, before I squat I always do hip openers to prepare my hips for the upcoming squat moves. The stretches are dynamic movements that take about 10–15 minutes at the start of the workout and they're an essential element.

Increased mobility will expand your range of motion, improve form and decrease the possibility of injury as well as reducing how stiff you feel after the workout. The problem with not taking the time to do these is that different parts of your body will end up over-compensating, just like in my case, where my ankles lacked the requisite mobility to safely perform squats or lunges without my knees and hips having to over-compensate. In the long run, you will slow down your progress if you lack a sufficient range of mobility. Even simple tasks will become harder, like bending down or going up the stairs. If you leave out these exercises, I will know, and I will hunt you down.

Mobility exercises

There are any number of mobility exercises out there that will help prime your muscles, supporting them in whatever workout you do and generally helping to keep stiffness at bay. Here are a few that I try to do most days. They should be applying pressure and feeling firm but not painful, so don't overdo it. Instead, ease yourself into each stretch. The more you practise, the more limber and flexible you'll feel. If your body is shouting 'Noooo!', don't go so deep into the stretch, as you'll only end up hurting yourself. I recommend using a yoga mat or a couple of towels underneath you, particularly for the exercises that put pressure on the knees.

Hips

Frog: Get onto all fours and slowly move both knees out to the sides. Ease into this stretch if it's new to you. Flex your ankles and push your feet out to the sides (it's the insides of your feet that should be against the floor). Again, move them out only to as far as they want to go (it will get further with time). Stretch your forearms out, placing them flat on the floor, palms down. Stay here for as long as is comfortable and when you're ready to release, do so slowly.

World's greatest stretch: Starting in a plank position, hop your right leg forward so it's level with your right hand, just outside of it. Enjoy this nice stretchy feeling for a moment before reaching your right hand up to the ceiling, pulling your shoulder back and opening across your chest. Hold for however long is comfortable and repeat on the other side.

Ankles

Kneeling ankle rocks: Kneeling down in front of a wall, lift your right knee and place your foot on the floor, with your toes a few inches away from the wall. Reach your palms out to the wall in front for support and slowly move your right knee towards the wall, going backwards and forwards for about 30 seconds. Switch and do the same on the other side.

Ankle release: Standing up, keeping your right ankle on the floor, flex the foot, pointing the toes towards the ceiling, holding for about 30–45 seconds and repeating several times. Switch to the other side. Hold on to a wall if you're struggling to balance.

Thoracic spine

Active child's pose: Begin on all fours and stretch your bum back towards your feet while keeping your arms stretched outwards and palms firmly on the floor. If you like, you can make this more dynamic by adding slow movement between the all fours and sitting back on your heels positions, repeating as many times as you like.

Cat to cow: On all fours, lift up your chest and face towards the ceiling, drawing your shoulders back. From here, move your face down to look at the floor between your hands and bring a gentle curve to your spine, rounding your upper back towards the ceiling. Flow gently between the poses.

Supine twists: Lying on a mat, bring both legs in towards your body with your palms on your shins. Keeping your back on the mat, roll your legs to the right (don't worry if they don't reach the floor), stay here for as long as is comfy and repeat on the other side for roughly the same about of time.

Shoulders

Prayer stretch: Get into an active child's pose and, keeping your feet together, move your knees to the side to make space for your body to fold over in between them. Bring your upper body down onto the floor, arms stretched out. Keeping your elbows and forehead on the ground (or on a block or even a big book, if that's more comfortable), lift up your hands, bringing the palms together like you are praying. Hang out here for as long as is comfortable.

Squatting

When you look at toddlers, you'll see their open hips and general stretchiness means they're often in a squat as they play with toys or mess about. They're completely comfortable in this natural resting seat – we all were until we became obsessed with sitting on chairs, making us more stiff as our muscles and joints became lazier, having to work less hard. It's really noticeable too if you travel to certain places in the world, like in Asia, where it's often the norm for all age groups to sit on the floor at mealtimes, usually cross-legged. It means that most people of all generations in those countries are much more limber than we, their European counterparts, are. We have forgotten these natural movements and spend way too much time being supported by our sofas, desk chairs and car seats. The downsides of this can be a host of health issues like back pain and postural problems. There have even been experiments where chairs were removed from school classrooms, the intention being to promote more focus in children and reduce shenanigans. Sitting down has been described as a worldwide epidemic. So, take every opportunity you can to *not* sit down. If you do need to sit, move frequently – fidget and stretch, get up and walk around every 30 minutes at the very least.

Squatting is where your body wants to be. Every day I try to sit in the bottom of a squat for ten minutes. I won't lie, it feels pretty punishing (sometimes I shed a tear through my clenched eyelids), but I built it up gradually, slowly eking out the time. I do it because it helps with back pain (which for me comes from imbalances in my body) and improves alignment between my hips, knees and thoracic spine.

Here's a quick guide to doing a deep squat. There are many slightly different ways that people squat, but this is mine. If at the start you can't do a squat without falling over, do it with a wall behind you to support you and your balance will gradually improve.

1. With your legs slightly further than hip-width apart, plant your feet firmly on the ground, being careful to distribute the weight evenly between both feet.
2. Bend your knees and keep them nicely parallel (rather than caving in towards each other).
3. Drop your bum as far as possible back and down towards the floor, going as low as you can.
4. Keep the spine aligned and pretty straight (don't round it) and the chest open, without the shoulders slumping.
5. Stretch your arms out at shoulder height, with your fingers stretched out and your palms parallel and facing each other. Keep the arms active and energised.

Give it a go every day. Ideally you'd want to be in this position for two minutes, but it may take a while to build up to that, so do what you can, holding it for slightly longer each time.

Useful mobility equipment

If you're joining a gym, you can check whether they have these items there, otherwise you might like to consider adding some of these to your gym bag.

Hockey ball/myofascial ball: This gives a deep-tissue massage, using your body weight to apply strong pressure.

Foam roller: This covers a greater surface area than the hockey ball so it's a less intense alternative for massage.

Peanut roller: A double-sided hockey ball, useful for working out the triceps and shins.

Thera Cane: I often use this hook-shaped massager while watching telly in the evening – it's great for getting into deep muscles.

Voodoo Floss: When wrapped tightly around muscles, this rubber compression band improves range, restores joint mechanics and unglues matted tissue.

Resistance bands (light and heavy): These are very important for stretching end-ranges and priming pre-workout.

Calisthenics and gymnastics

These are two other disciplines that really aid and facilitate good mobility that I want to give a shout-out to. Firstly, calisthenics, from the Greek *kalos* and *sthenos*, meaning beauty and strength, which sum up it up pretty well in my opinion. This really is a beautiful and elegant style of training – two adjectives never before associated with me. While bodybuilding is mostly about aesthetics – making the muscles look big and bulky – with calisthenics it's all about how functional they are. Calisthenics takes a person through a series of exercises that promote strength, flexibility, endurance, balance and control. It moves your body through different plains and enables range of motion. Practising calisthenics will give you mastery of your body weight; you'll be lean and mean, without any excess bulk weighing you down. There's no need to blow what you'd set aside for council tax on any equipment, either. All you need is the ground you walk on and some outdoor bars, which, depending on your area, you may well find in an outdoor gym in a park (otherwise hit up the monkey bars in a playground. Joking! Or am I . . . ?). If worst comes to worst, you can even use a wall. If at any point you add weights, however, it no longer falls into the calisthenics category, but becomes resistance training instead.

Similarly, gymnastics is all about the beauty of movement – moving the body as it's designed to. It celebrates the flexibility of the joints and skeleton rather than individual muscles. Gymnasts have amazing core strength and posture, with a reverence of the spine as a central source of strength in the body. They are ridiculously skilled athletes, able to hold positions for a seriously impressive amount of time. Have you ever seen a picture or video of someone holding on to a vertical bar with their hands and their whole body stretched out, floating in the air, all in line parallel to the ground? It looks more like levitation than anything a human might be capable of.

Both types of training will bring you overall strength by building muscle mass. Gymnastics is gym-based, whereas calisthenics uses the world outside as its gym – which is one reason why some prefer one over the other.

I've dabbled in a bit of bar work, but the reason I'm not a fully-fledged gymnast or calisthitian (it's a word, okay?) is because you can't really get ridiculously big and powerful doing this type of training alone; there's a threshold for how far you can develop within it. I get that not everyone wants to be a mutant, and that's okay (I suppose). Remember the type 1 and 2 muscle fibres? (See page 63 if you need a refresher.) If you spend hours walking or jogging every day, you'd think you'd be owed mega muscles, given the time you're putting in. Alas, no; you'll be super-fit in the endurance sense but not muscly, because the exercise gives your type 1 fibres a great workout but doesn't reach as far as type 2. Calisthenics and gymnastics are a bit like that, in the sense that you'll condition yourself to get better, but after a certain point your body won't adapt further because no new stimulus has been introduced. Because you use your own body weight as resistance, it's not as simple as adding extra resistance as you might do when lifting free weights, increasing the load over time.

If you're interested in finding out more about calisthenics or gymnastics, try to get to a local club and, in the first instance, before you invest in that leotard, ask if you can observe a class or training session to give you a sense of what's involved. Learning these disciplines under the guidance of experts is the way to go.

GYMNASTICS AND CALISTHENICS

What gymnastics and calisthenics deliver: Build functional strength and improve flexibility, balance and coordination.

Why they work: They encourage good alignment and build whole-body strength using body weight as resistance.

Physique: Lean and toned.

Pros: Both disciplines help build overall fitness and strength, and there's a good social element as they tend to be done in groups. They also rely on significant mental focus.

Cons: Like many sports, there are cases of extremes, with people pushing themselves too far and causing themselves injury. Both gymnastics and calisthenics should be practised under expert supervision.

Equipment: Gymnastics relies on quite a bit of kit, including balance beams, pulley rings, horses and spring floors. Calisthenics uses equipment like pull-up bars, resistance bands and pulley rings.

Importance of technique: Good positioning and alignment will help you make progress and prevent injury.

LIFT

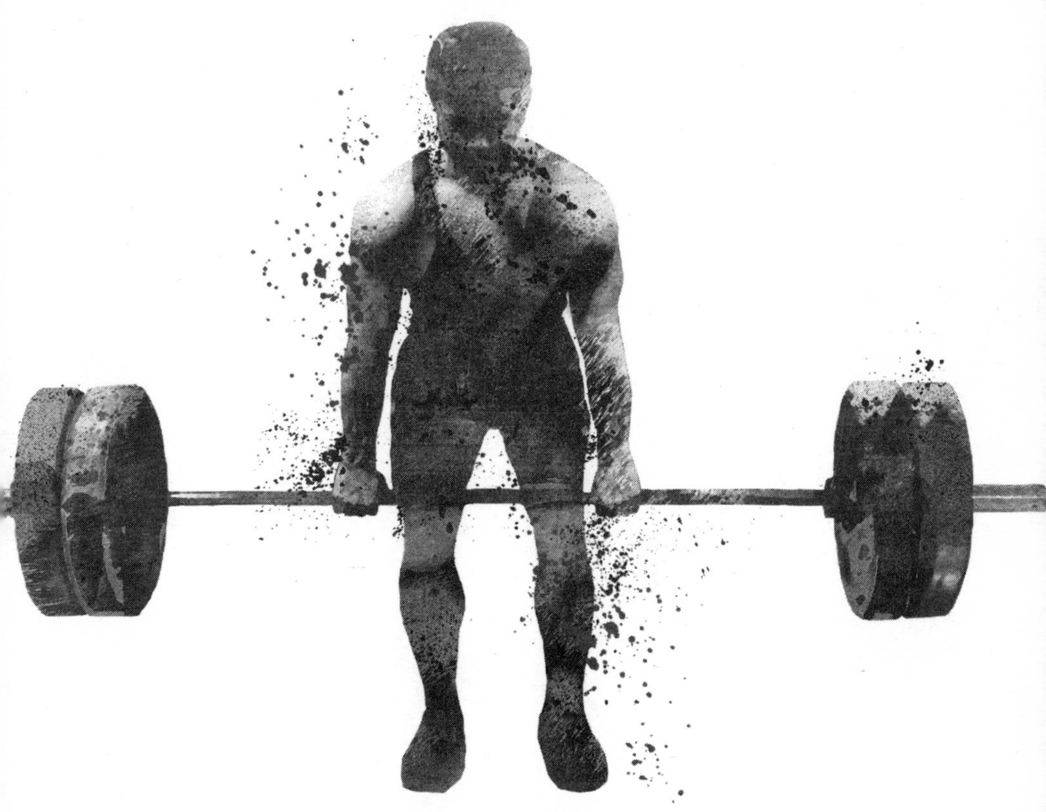

JUST LIKE IN the previous sections, I have some cracking workouts here to get you lifting. But before you all throw the book down and run to find a bench press, there's some info I want to give you. Even though I'm like a Labrador who always wants to get stuck into something straight away (panting, sniffing, licking myself etc.), I reckon it might do you good to first familiarise yourself with some of the science behind weightlifting (even if you've been lifting for ages), because it *will* benefit your progress.

I often meet people who can't face exercise because they find it boring. (Heathens!) When I give them a healthy bit of banter (verbal abuse) about such an outrageous statement, it almost always emerges that the only exercise they've tried is cardio-based. Sometimes this is a hangover from school days, where PE lessons were all about running (or communal showers). So, if cardio doesn't appeal right now, let me show you the bright lights of strength training using weights. Don't be put off by the idea that lifting weights is a go-big-or-go-home sport – I promise you it's not. You can definitely be both a hardcore balls-to-the-wall type or more of a part-timer who likes to lift a bit at the weekend. Gone are the days when it was only about bulking up for that *lads, lads, lads* trip to Magaluf, strutting down the beach in the hope of getting some unholy boom-boom time. Fortunately, it has moved beyond that stereotype, and is becoming popular with all kinds of people looking to boost their health. An element of resistance training should be part of everyone's – young or old, male or female – routine, because:

- It burns calories both during and after the workout, boosting your metabolism and helping sustain a healthy weight.
- It can help increase bone mass and prevent diseases like osteoporosis.
- It helps prevent injury, as you'll build more muscle tissue.
- As with exercise in general, it can boost your mood, reduce stress and improve your overall wellbeing.

We've looked at some disciplines that use body weight for strength training, such as gymnastics, plyometrics and yoga, but here it's all about the iron. There are many different types of weightlifting that will appeal to people for different reasons. In this section we'll be looking at bodybuilding and powerlifting, because I think they offer an excellent foundation for learning about strength, and they are good starting points from which you can branch out if you want to explore another strand, such as Strongman/woman.

The plans I give a bit later on for weightlifting can all be carried out in a regular high-street gym. If you decide to mix it up further and take lifting to a pretty serious level, you might want to consider going to a specialist lifters' gym, where there will be more niche equipment available. If you're picturing saunas and pitchers of water with cucumbers floating in them, I'm afraid they're more like Hades' underworld than the Elysian fields. Lifters' gyms are all about getting shit done. They're often relatively cheap to join but not always especially cheerful! I love them, though; there's no dicking around by the smoothie bar – everyone is focused on pushing themselves to the max, which spurs me on.

Tear, eat, rest, repeat

Weightlifting. If the word alone makes you feel a bit 'wtf . . .?', just remember that weightlifting extends far beyond the four walls of your gym, and you're probably already doing lots of it on a day-to-day basis. Carrying your laundry basket out to the washing line? Weightlifting. Lifting your kid out of the car seat? Weightlifting. Bringing your shopping bags out of the supermarket? Weightlifting. All this is a good start if you want to progress to machine weights at the gym and then on to free weights.

I always recommend gym newbies begin with an element of bodybuilding even if they don't want it to be their main focus. If you've been inactive, the first port of call will be for you to switch on your motor units (see page 64), and bodybuilding will help activate these dormant cells. Essentially, you're firing up the central nervous system, which will help support your training. This is why, if you're a beginner, you should focus on getting stronger overall. You'll notice the biggest change at the start of your training programme because you'll be activating motor units at a rapid pace. Remember, you'll also be burning calories both during and after a session, unlike many aerobic-only regimes, so it's a good option if you want to lose some body fat. Lifting defies gravity and the buzz you get from it is addictive – which is why weightlifters keep coming back for more.

People are often surprised to learn how many technical

considerations there are in relation to weightlifting (and it's why this section of the book is quite long). It's definitely not just a case of rocking up to the gym and going at it hammer and tongs. Of course, you do see people doing that and it spells disaster for their progress and increases their potential to cause damage to themselves. It's essential to understand how your body is working away to support your training so that you can harness these physiological processes according to your goals. If you have been giving the training your all and you haven't been seeing the results you were expecting, it may be that you haven't considered some of the factors coming up.

Adaptation

Periodisation training – and there are many forms of it in this book – is the term that describes workouts that frequently change up the movements you do. If you follow the same workout routine day in, day out, a point will come where you plateau – and this is true for any exercise you do. You won't get stronger and you may overwork yourself, leading to muscle or CNS fatigue. By changing it up, whether that's every session or every few weeks, you will target different muscle groups and give yourself adequate time to recover. Think of it as being like when you are at work – you can't just focus on the same task for eight hours; you'd find yourself getting more distracted, glancing at your phone, staring out the window, as your productivity continues to wane.

Progression and overload

The harder you work your body, the more it develops, meaning that if you push yourself a little harder each session, you'll be triggering an overload. This is where the body gets used to practising a particular exercise through repetition, and becomes stronger as a result. A muscle adaptation sees stress being put on a muscle, which it then adapts to. For example, exercises that work the tendons make them more efficient and better able to accommodate exercise. So, if you're a runner training for a 10k, each week at least one of your runs might get a bit longer, and when applied to weightlifting, each week you might be lifting a little more weight or doing more reps or sets than the week before. Six to twelve reps is prime for building muscle fibres, whereas if you go above twelve, it's likely to become more endurance-based, so just be mindful of that.

To facilitate progressive overload, rest is vital, because if you've pushed yourself beyond comfortable capacity, it's when you rest after the training session that the muscles build. We looked at hypertrophy a little earlier on (this is the increase in muscle cells through exercise through damage and repair) and weightlifting is one of the most prominent ways of achieving it, as it'll make your muscles bigger and more conditioned. To maintain muscle mass and bone density, we need to push ourselves beyond our comfort levels at least a couple of times a week (as is the case with every type of exercise, not just lifting). As I alternate my workout between four weeks of bodybuilding and four weeks of powerlifting, it means I can test my previous month's workout to see that it had the effects it was meant to – basically checking to see if I have successfully overloaded my system and become stronger.

It's not all about beating the shit out of yourself, though; progressive overload gains can be made through some small, sometimes subtle increases. For example, if you are trying to ensure you achieve progressive overload but don't want to lift heavier weights, another muscle stimulus would be changing up your workout with a few weeks of volume training (i.e. sets × reps × weight = volume). The best bodybuilders I know go by how they feel and how the muscles feel, rather than the numbers written on the weights they're lifting.

Lifting and the CNS

Yep, I'm talking about the central nervous system again, because it comes into its own with certain elements of lifting. Depending on the type you're doing, it will have a different impact on your nervous system, and you don't want to get your signals crossed (literally).

The CNS is responsible for muscle contractions. Imagine you are picking up a stick; well, this happens because your brain sends signals via neurons to your hand. You'll pick up a small stick using a corresponding amount of strength. Let's say that stick has become a larger, heavier branch; your brain increases the level of motor units it sends your arm in order for you to lift it. Your brain might also send signals to your other arm to help brace the lifting arm. It might help you plant your feet, sending strength up through your legs and core, priming the whole body to lift the branch.

Bodybuilding, which focuses on slow, repetitive movements like isolation curls, fatigues rather than stimulates the nervous system, because your brain is mostly sending signals just to your arm and not much more than that. This can sometimes mean that bodybuilders who look huge are actually not super-strong, relatively speaking; they've increased the size of the muscles without increasing the strength of them. Powerlifters, on the other hand, often look smaller than bodybuilders but because powerlifting really fires up the CNS, they have more strength.

Strategic rest

Later on in the book, I talk about how vital it is to get enough shut-eye if you are training, as it's during sleep that your body is able to redirect energy into repairing itself. Think of all those microtears in the muscle that have occurred during training which need to mend. On top of that, you won't feel particularly motivated to exercise if you're knackered. Skip ahead to page 292 for some tips on maximising Zzzs.

The other essential rest is the type that breaks up your workout. You are resting to get the best out of your regime, rather than just for the fun of a quick chit-chat with your workout buddy (though a bit of bantz is a bonus). Resting is a way of changing up the stimulus in order to shock the body, and depending on the type of exercise you're doing (e.g. high-intensity interval training or different types of weightlifting), there will be different strategies for rest. In powerlifting, for example, you might have a relatively short rest period of 30–45 seconds when lifting lighter weights or doing isolation exercises, and then increasing the rest period when using heavier weights and compound-based exercises. This will mean you'll be changing up the stimulus and therefore avoiding a plateau.

When you're lifting, if you're not resting for a minimum

of 30 seconds between sets, you're doing cardio with weights rather than resistance. There's nothing wrong with that, so long as you know what you're doing! If you're not giving your body recovery time to allow the lactate to disperse, then it becomes your aerobic system that you're working. This is often the reason at play when people aren't making the progress they'd aimed for. They think they're doing themselves a favour by pushing it to the max but they're unwittingly working another system in the body, which is taking progress away from the area they actually want to develop.

Inside our muscles cells is a small store of adenosine triphosphate (ATP) and creatine phosphate (CP), enough to power a couple of seconds of high-intensity movement. CP comes into effect very quickly, taking over from the ATP, to continue powering the muscle contraction and relaxation. We use ATP constantly, even in sleep.

The CNS also needs rest. Overdoing volume or intensity can tire it out and affect your performance, so if you're noticing you're a bit lacklustre at the gym, and your lifts are lacking precision and energy, it might be time to try to reboot the CNS. Do so by switching up your gym sessions and, if you're feeling generally frazzled, try to take some time out to slow down. If you are barely keeping up on the treadmill of life combined with hitting it hard fitness-wise, you might be burning out your CNS.

Mind to muscle (MTM)

Bodybuilding and yoga aren't famed for their similarities, but they have more in common than you think. Eastern philosophy has long since linked the body and mind (thank you,

Karate Kid, for everything you have taught me), but it seems to have taken us much longer in the West. Seeing our bodies as a single entity, with the mind impacting on the body and vice versa, should be obvious. If one isn't feeling good, it's likely the other will soon follow suit.

So, the process of mind to muscle is a way of building muscle by using a bit of mindfulness. It all sounds a bit New Age, but it is an ingrained part of professional weightlifting, particularly in powerlifting and Olympic lifting. It involves every movement within a lift being really considered, as you try to think deliberately about what every muscle is doing, engaging every part of the body that is supporting the movement. So, using slow, controlled movements versus faster ones increases muscle fibres and can make two 15s feel like 40s, so it works in tandem with the amount of time the muscle is under tension. It's an amazing thing that just thinking about every movement makes the lift more challenging.

The question of volume (how much weight you're lifting) versus intensity (for how many reps or sets) is one that everyone has a different opinion on. It can be very tempting to want to focus more on the weight, bashing out the reps just to get it done and to say you can lift X amount, and I have certainly been caught up in this ego mindset in the past. What about lifting less but spending more time doing so? If I am squatting with 60kg on my back/shoulders, thinking about every subtle movement – the form of my torso, the angle of my thighs to knees, the positioning of my head – it'll be harder than ten fast reps (*boom, boom, boom!*) of squatting with twice the weight. The next time you're doing a pull-up on a bar, concentrate on your biceps, then change it up on the next rep and bring the focus to the lats, then, for the next rep, send more energy to your traps. Working in this way targets specific motor units, paving the way for hypertrophy.

The very best bodybuilders approach their training with mind to muscle at the forefront, interspersing their fast lifts with controlled MTM movements. If you are already a seasoned lifter and have only been doing explosive fast lifting, start including mind-to-muscle lifting and you'll see massive growth, as the change will shock your body.

Time under tension (TUT) and tempo

As we know, by adjusting the stimulus, your body becomes stronger as metabolic stress keeps your body on the gain train. Another way to build muscle is to consider time under tension (the time that the muscle is under stress) and eccentric loading in particular (fast-forward to page 210 for more on contractions). If I'm working with someone who is new to resistance training, I often start them out with pull-ups. At the beginning I'll probably need to lift them up to the bar and they may or may not be able to hold their body weight, gripping onto the bar for a few seconds before jumping down. Without even pulling up, this process will build muscles in their lats. After a few sessions, they'll hold the bar for slightly longer (extending the time under tension), each week getting stronger. It matters more to hold your eccentric and isometric (the pause during a lift) parts for longer to build muscle than the heaviness of the weight (obviously you need some resistance – somewhere in between a toilet roll and a pony).

Another way to mix up the stimulus is by playing around with the tempo with which you move the weights. The 4-2-2 speed is a prime method for building muscle and refers to the seconds you hold each move for, where the muscle is under tension – for example, lowering the bar slowly to your chest for four seconds, resting for two seconds and pushing it out for two seconds.

Metabolic stress and mechanical tension

These are theories in weight training about how the body most efficiently damages and, in turn, builds muscle. Boffins of the bodybuilding scene debate which is the more effective way to gain muscle mass, with the general consensus veering towards mechanical tension being superior. I consulted 'Glute Guy' Dr Bret Contreras, bodybuilding pro, sports scientist and all-round muscle expert, for his two cents on the subject. He explained that there's still a lot we don't know about exactly what's going on when a muscle is activated, as the science behind building muscle and cell swelling is still emerging.

Metabolic stress (also called the pump) is used in bodybuilding and is often associated with higher reps and shorter rest periods. With metabolic stress, there's still always some mechanical tension at play because when you put increased tension on the muscle, even with lighter loads, that leads to more muscle growth. The harder you tense, the more tension you create. In the case of higher reps, you'll never have as much absolute tension on the muscle at any one point, but throughout the set, all the fibres get activated sufficiently – assuming you push the set hard and go to failure (i.e. doing as many reps as you possibly can). As you fatigue, muscle activation goes up, so if you have a 20-rep set, during the first five reps you won't have that higher muscle activation, but over the last five reps, muscle activation goes way up. This is due to fatigue, so all the fibres do end up getting sufficient tension to stimulate hypertrophy, meaning higher reps will lead to mechanical tension.

Mechanical tension is utilised more in powerlifting and it's the flex of the muscle that creates the tension within it. Imagine there's a car over-turned in the street and you have to use superhuman strength to roll it back over. If there are five muscle fibres you use to push the car, the first three are the slow-twitch ones, which give smaller, sustained movements, and then the two fast-twitch ones come into use when you need greater force. If your body can't push the car with just one hand, you would naturally bring in your second hand to help, and you'd also start bracing your core. The fast-twitch fibres get going when you really exert yourself, so the better your ability to recruit high-twitch fibres, the better the hypertrophy response. The first time you attempt to push the car, it's going to be really difficult, if not impossible, but each time you try it gets easier, because each time your body has adapted and your muscles have got bigger and stronger – provided you have rested and eaten well (not a lot of gains will be made if you prop up the bar after every gym session!).

There was a study that looked at both approaches, monitoring powerlifters using mechanical tension and bodybuilders drawing on metabolic stress. Both groups had to lift 300kg in poundage in a bicep curl. The powerlifters approached the task by lifting 100kg over 3 reps, which took them 30 minutes; the bodybuilders did 30kg over 10 reps, which took them 10 minutes to complete, i.e. a higher number of reps over a much quicker timeframe. After eight weeks, there was no difference in hypertrophy response in either approach, but the powerlifters became slightly stronger. In the powerlifters' mechanical tension method (doing 3 reps at a higher weight) there was more fatigue and injury, and these injuries prevented longer-term progress. What this suggests is that there's no ideal rep range to build muscle; even if you're doing 12–15 reps, you'll be developing your slow-twitch fibres, meaning you'll be able to lift for longer. It's through periodisation training that you'll build up your lactate threshold, to stop plateaus.

Load, velocity, mind to muscle

With mechanical tension, if you're doing an 80% load of your 1 rep max, you'll only recruit four of the five muscle fibres. But if you have a 70% load and you try to pull the weight up hard and fast, you'll recruit that fifth fibre, so the load doesn't always have to be at its highest to get to it, so long as there's velocity. Go one step further to lift with a mind-to-muscle approach, activating the muscle in a conscious and deliberate way, as well as lifting the weights. This is metabolic stress combined with mechanical tension. Just keep in mind that the more motor units are recruited, the stronger you'll be in the long run.

mTOR pathway (mammalian target of rapamycin): This is one of the body's energy sensors and cell signals that, when activated, stimulates hypertrophy, leading to muscle growth through protein synthesis. Its signalling pathway is a regulator of metabolism and growth, and one of the ways it's activated is through the release of ATP.

Delayed onset muscle soreness (DOMS)

This is the soreness you feel in your muscles and temporary reduction in strength, caused by muscle inflammation, which often peaks around 24–72 hours after a hardcore workout. While uncomfortable, it can also feel very satisfying to know you've pushed yourself hard. But don't be fooled – you can still damage the muscle (i.e. tear fibres leading to muscle growth) and it won't necessarily be sore. So, don't strive for soreness, because you can be building muscle without pain later on; pain shouldn't be used as an assessment of how much the muscle is growing. The trick to knowing if you're gaining strength is good programming as well as how quickly you recover before you can use that muscle again. You don't need to have the thrash-yourself bodybuilder mentality to make gains. Having lectured you on that, I've got to say I can be terrible for trying to destroy myself when I train. I know I shouldn't but I can't help myself. Just know that even if you feel like you've woken up in prison with Mike Tyson hanging out the back of you, it doesn't necessarily mean that session has been more productive than one where you've worked out at a less intense pace.

Ways to change up the stimulus

- Tempo training: Playing around with time under tension – alternate fast, explosive lifting using heavier weights with slower, controlled ones using lighter weights
- Alternate the types of training you do every eight weeks (for example, I do four weeks of bodybuilding followed by four weeks of powerlifting)

- Alternating sets, reps and weight volume
- Increasing your range of motion (see below)
- Perfecting your technique using mind to muscle
- Eccentric loading (controlling the lengthening phase of each repetition)
- Changing up the rest periods
- Supersets and giant sets
- Partial reps
- Taking it to failure

Range of motion (ROM)

The degree to which your joints move when flexing or extending reflects your range of motion. And it's a vital (but often overlooked) part of weightlifting because if your range of motion is limited, your body won't be able to adequately support the movements you do. Think of ROM as building a body that's specific to the sport you're doing, helping you excel. It's important to also look at flexibility here because this stems from soft tissue like muscles and tendons, and being more flexible enables greater range of motion. Some people are born with Stretch Armstrong limbs that seem to bend every which way (they must be dynamite in the sack), but other poor fools (me) have to work on it. I was a bollocks for neglecting these in my years as a footballer and rugby player. Like a lot of lifters, I saw them as an optional extra that took a bit of time and wouldn't make a huge amount of difference – back then I'd have rather spent every available minute in the 'doing' rather than the 'preparing'. It's only relatively recently that I have started investing the energy in it, and it's paid off, because I am stronger and more flexible as a result.

Your range of motion can change depending on whether you have an injury or another condition, and it may become limited either temporarily or more permanently. But focusing on your ROM, through doing exercises that mobilise your joints, you can also prevent injury.

Different strands of weightlifting utilise ROM in various ways. If you've ever watched Olympic lifting on telly, you'll see they need to move as efficiently as possible, so their range of motion works hard to support their technique. They arch their feet, using them as anchors, which then gives an arch in the back, and they then squeeze their shoulders together to shorten their range of motion as they lift the bar. One of the ways they train is by perfecting their squat position with a massive range of motion. When they're at the bottom of a snatch, that's their range of motion at its deepest and most mobile (if I attempted an overhead squat in that position my spine would probably burst out of my skin).

So, you can see from observing them how a solid range of motion enables a good form. When you start any weight-lifting, focusing on form is essential both to support your movements and also to prevent injury. On top of that, when you practise good form and are deliberate about your technique, once it's ingrained it becomes automatic and you'll do it without even thinking about it (and the same is true if you practise a bad technique). If you're bodybuilding, you'll also be using mobility to recruit muscle fibres. So if you are in a 90° squat lifting 100kg, you'll be better off dropping that weight to 90kg and trying to improve your mobility so that you bring your arse lower (or 'ass to grass' if you speak meathead). This way you'll be recruiting more muscle fibres and so muscle-building potential will be higher, even though you're lifting a lower amount. Once you're more mobile, you can increase the weight again and you should find that your movements are so much more efficient.

I'm evangelical about maximising ROM, so read my mobility drills on page 177 where I bore you some more.

Make Love to Thy Barbell

Before you get lifting using the plans coming up, keep the following info in mind.

Training regimes

There are different approaches to training, but once you get beyond beginner level, I'm a big believer in targeting just a couple of muscle groups per session on rotation, rather than doing a full-body workout each time.

'Push, Pull, Legs' is a classic routine that divides the body into three parts and you exercise each part in its own workout, alternating between each one. 'Push' focuses on the upper body, pushing the muscles of the shoulders, chest and triceps. 'Pull' is when you work the upper body's pulling muscles: the back and biceps. 'Legs' is all about the lower body, i.e. the glutes, quads, hamstrings and calves. The abdominals can be touched in any exercises at any time. The other type you might have heard of is what's called 'The Bro-Split', which targets one or two muscle groups per workout; for example, it might be back and biceps one day, chest and triceps the next.

Compartmentalising in this way allows the muscles to recover between sessions, and for gym freaks (like myself!) it means you can go to the gym five or six days a week if you want to. It's an efficient way of moving your body and you see the effects. You'll notice that in the workouts I set out later on I don't specify the weights you should be using, as this will be individual to your current strength and goals.

Reps, sets and time under tension (TUT)

Reps (meaning repetitions) are the backbone of strength training; they're the number of times you repeat a certain exercise, like a squat or a pull-up. A set is a group of repetitions. The number of reps you perform versus the resistance you're using is a bit of a formula, and depending on this formula it will have a different impact on the body and how quickly you progress. The number of reps will determine how many sets you do as well as the rest period, so the higher number of reps, the lower the sets will be. The idea is that you increase the number of reps and/or sets as your body gets used to them so that you are always progressing, challenging your body so that it gets stronger. Time under tension is however long the muscles are under strain during a particular movement. It's the tension that forces the muscle to contract and in turn it is what makes it stronger over time. You can play around with the time your muscles are under tension depending on what you want to achieve.

The rep max

This is the maximum amount of weight you can lift for one repetition, which is a way of measuring how strong you are. If you're lifting weights at an intermediate level, it's a good test to do. A simple way to find your one rep max (or 1RM) is to get someone to spot you at the gym and, on the bench press, gradually increase the weights you lift until you come to the heaviest you can lift for one repetition. If you're at a loose end, this can actually be a superb spectator sport when you spot an egolifter at the gym attempting a 1RM way beyond their rep range – pull up a pew and grab a bag of popcorn, because you're about to see the bar just about rise up and then pluuuuuuuuummet down. RIP.

If you follow my advanced plans for bodybuilding, you'll see that I suggest a percentage of your rep max. This percentage determines how much you should be lifting for your other rep ranges, so it means you can lift at a level inkeeping with your current strength and adjust it as you progress. When you are bodybuilding and you have your 1RM, you should be working to 90% of your 1RM; this is your training rep max, rather than your competition rep max. So my 1 rep competition max might be 340kg, but my training rep max would be 320kg.

Grip strength

How firmly you can hold onto an object is one of the ways used to determine overall muscular strength by measuring the tension created in the forearm when gripping, also taking into account the weight of the object. Gripping draws on the muscles in the forearm, hand, wrist and fingers. With a strong grip you can lift heavier weights, especially when you are doing pulling movements. It can also aid your endurance and is generally helpful with everyday tasks as well as in exercise like powerlifting, climbing or racket-based sports. Lifting weights will naturally develop your grip strength.

Contractions

Don't worry, I'm not suggesting you go into spontaneous labour here. These types of contractions are the three main parts of every resistance training exercise you do. The different phases of a lift put muscles under varying periods of strain, which results in extensive muscle breakdown, leading to maximum growth.

Concentric: This is the shortening of the muscles and tends to be the first part of your lift when following the upcoming plans. For example, this would be the start of a deadlift, when you're bringing it up off the floor or coming up to a sit-up position.

Isometric: This is the holding of weight in one spot, where the lift pauses halfway (such as coming halfway up in a deadlift) and the muscle isn't moving, and it's usually the toughest part of the lift. Some exercises naturally include a pause moment and you can add them in to others.

Eccentric: This is the lengthening of the muscle, using the aid of gravity, such as lowering yourself down from a pull-up bar, and it has the maximum potential for strengthening the muscles, tendons and ligaments. Creating more tension in the lengthening of the muscle also recruits more motor units.

BODYBUILDING

> 'On the surface bodybuilding is about sculpting and improving the physique. However, it's actually a 24-hour-a-day job – you need to train hard, eat properly for your goals, manage stress and get adequate sleep in order to achieve your best body. The diligence and consistency required to do so will improve your work ethic, provide structure to your day, and ultimately transfer over to other areas in your life.'
>
> DR BRET CONTRERAS, WORLD-LEADING HYPERTROPHY EXPERT

Picture some of the gods from mythology, like Atlas, doomed to hold the heavens on his shoulders for eternity. Atlas, the poor fucker, punished with lugging the weight of the world around but . . . don't worry! Look at those triceps, lats and traps! In every depiction we see of Atlas, he has the physique of a bodybuilder – chiselled, muscular and with no body fat to speak of. It's the idealised version of humanity, one that you see repeated in works of art since the beginning of time; the 'perfect' form. When I was a kid I used to love watching *Dragon Ball Z*, where the main character Piccolo was a super-ripped cartoon figure. I remember thinking, 'Wow, how do I get a body like that?!' It was only years later, when I started hitting the gym myself, that I released my screen idol had the frame of a bodybuilder, and weirdly this ideal had lodged itself in my consciousness.

Before we get into the meaty stuff, I want to clarify here the type of bodybuilding I'll be talking about, because there is a scale. If you are picturing a shiny, grinning Arnie from the '70s wearing gold pants on a podium, all waxed and oiled, move along, because that's a different discipline. That is professional bodybuilding, which is more about making the body look a certain way, like shrinking the waist and getting the quad symmetry. So, you might be relieved to hear I am not about to dictate a plan that will have you reaching for a thong and the spray tan.

The bodybuilding I'm talking about is a form of resistance training that forms the foundations for so many sports. In essence, it's about making your body strong, usually by focusing on specific areas, one at one time, so that it can adapt to whatever discipline you throw at it. Professional footballers, swimmers, tennis players – the list goes on – will all do some bodybuilding in the gym as part of a wider training programme. There are so many benefits that come with this type of strength training (see page 228), and we should all be doing some of it. Traditionally bodybuilding has been dominated by men in their twenties and thirties but more recently there has been more take-up by women and also older people. It can be particularly beneficial for the latter, in fact, as it's thought it can help with general aches and pains and the symptoms of conditions like osteoporosis and arthritis, and even help reduce the risk of developing them in the first place, as well as boosting mental health and general wellbeing.

It may be that you only follow my beginner's plan, or perhaps take it up to intermediate level 1. This will give you an incredible foundation for strength, and will then boost your performance in other sports. On the other hand, you might realise bodybuilding is your 'thing' and work your way through to the advanced workouts.

Bodybuilding works by building muscle through slow repetition, where the muscle spends more time under tension and becomes stronger as a consequence. Remember those fast-twitch muscle fibres from your physiology lesson earlier (see page 63)? These are the ones that support short and powerful movements like lifting a heavy weight. Muscles continue to build after the workout, which is why rest is so important, as it's during the downtime that protein synthesis repairs the muscle damage and glycogen can be replenished. If you follow my plan but are not being strategic about rest, you're going to be wasting your time.

All the information and workout plans are targeted at both women and men. I have often trained women who start out saying they don't want to do any weightlifting because they don't want to get 'too big', and I'm always quick to suggest just trying it and seeing how they feel after a few weeks. There sometimes seems to be a fear about the scales, especially for those – women and men – who want to lose a little weight and generally tone up. After four to six weeks of bodybuilding, someone might gain 3–4kg and they'll feel incredible. Tricep exercises during chest sessions have conditioned the upper body, which is an area many women, in particular, I've worked with are keen to target. The result is that after a month or so, the person is more toned and feels more comfortable in their clothes and more energetic, and feels empowered by the whole process. Result. But then they go and weigh themselves, and it turns out they haven't shed the pounds they'd originally been hoping to (they've maybe even gained a couple), and they feel disheartened after all their hard work. This is why the scales do not tell the whole story and shouldn't be used at all in situations like this. They often only serve to feed into a negative mindset (particularly for women, in my experience of being a PT) that progress is all based on the number on the scales going down. It's hardly surprising that many women feel like this, given the media portrayal of skinny as an ideal to aspire to. It's fuels a mental barrier around weight training, even for some women who are feeling and looking incredible off the back of it. So, I am telling you: get rid of the scales when you start this type of training and instead focus on how you feel!

Bodybuilding requires the acid and lactate systems to work in unison – by putting the muscles under stress, lactate builds, and this is what helps the muscles to grow. This is why lifting combined with short rest periods in between keeps the lactate in the muscles, allowing them to swell. As the weeks go on, if you want to make headway, you should be pushing yourself to get to the next step, embracing progressive overload, which will mean less rest between sets, using heavier weights, sustaining longer eccentric and isometric holds, and increasing reps and/or sets.

Whether bodybuilding is going to be your main fitness focus or if you're using it to build strength in conjunction with another type of training, these plans will get you results.

> 'When it comes to preparing for a show, not only is it you versus the other competitors on stage, it's you versus you 24 hours a day. It takes a different type of discipline and

commitment to do the work when the only person watching is the guy in the mirror staring back at you! There is no fooling that guy because he actually knows how hard you are working . . . and how much you really want it.'

SHAUN STAFFORD, TWO-TIME WBFF PHYSIQUE WORLD CHAMPION

Beginner's Workout

This is a full-body workout, containing five key compound lifts, to be done two to three times a week (leaving one to two days between sessions). It's the plan I'd give to someone flying solo at the gym, without a personal trainer. You'll see for Week 1 I haven't specified the number of reps, and this is because in the first instance you need to establish your baseline, by finding out how strong you are. So, do what you can, but you should find three sets of 12–15 reps a struggle. It may be that you achieve a good number of reps on the first set you do, but don't manage it on the next set – that's okay! Make a note on your phone to keep track of exactly what you've done, and compare these figures week on week. You'll start to notice progress after the first week or two.

If you are new to the gym, it's important to have an induction where a PT talks you through the different machines and shows you how to use them. Get them to earn their keep by observing your technique, as it's essential to learn the correct moves to prevent injury, particularly when using free weights. Don't be a buffoon by leaping on blind.

Lingo

Push, Pull, Legs (see page 207 for a refresher)

- Reps (repetitions): the number of times you repeat the exercise
- Sets: the groups of repetitions
- AMRAP: as many reps as possible
- %: percentage of your repetition max (see page 209 for more info)

WEEK 1

You are easing in this week, so just rep as many times as you can. Be sure to ask a trainer at the gym to show you how these machines work and to observe you when you first go on.

	EXERCISE	***SETS***
Push	Chest press machine	3
Legs	Leg press machine	3
Back	Lateral pulldowns	3
Legs	Leg curls	3
Shoulders	Shoulder press machine	3

WEEK 2

	EXERCISE	***REPS***	***SETS***
Day 1: Push	Chest press machine	12	4
	Incline press machine	12	4
	Shoulder press machine	12	4
	Peck deck machine	12	3
	Tricep pushdown (on the wires)	12	3
Day 2: Pull	Lateral pulldown	12	4
	Low row machine	12	4
	Reverse fly machine	12	3
	Dumbbell lateral raises	12	3
	Dumbbell bicep curls	12	3
Day 3: Legs	Leg extension machine	12	4
	Leg curl machine	12	4
	Leg press machine	12	4
	Calf raise machine	12	4

WEEK 3

When you get to Week 3, you can start thinking about incorporating free weights, changing up some of the compound lifts you've been doing for free-weight exercises. You'll follow Push, Pull, Legs on repeat, until you reach intermediate level, where you add more focus to other parts of the body like the chest, back and shoulders.

Here are some swaps to make:

Leg press machine – barbell squats
Leg curl machine – Romanian deadlifts
Chest press machine – dumbbell or barbell bench press
Low row machine – barbell bent-over row
Smith machine – barbell or dumbbell squat

This is the time when you need to start watching your imbalances to see if you have the stability and mobility needed to perform exercises efficiently. For example, you may find you don't yet have the ankle or hip manoeuvrability required, which is where mobility exercises come in (see page 179). As a beginner, you'll need to start looking at your movement mechanics to ensure your form is spot on – both to get the most from the exercise you're doing as well as preventing injury. If you don't feel confident assessing your form, ask one of the gym's trainers to observe your movements. Everyone makes mistakes at the start, so don't feel you have to know it all, as that's when I often see injuries happen. We need to push ourselves out of our comfort zone, but you can do so while going at your own pace (no, that's not a contradiction!). Respect your body and the speed at which it's adapting to these new exercises; it will be different for everyone. So, stick to the machine weights until you're comfortable tackling the free weights. It's important to learn to tap into how your body is progressing and what it needs both to be challenged and taken care of.

Intermediate Level 1 Workout

After about three or four weeks of the beginner's training, you can start thinking about cranking it up a notch. As you progress to this level, once again there's a certain amount of trial and error at the start to ascertain your strength, and that will determine how heavy the weights you use are. When you're trying these exercises for the first time, be sure to ask a PT at the gym to talk you through these movements and to observe you doing them so that they can give you pointers. Staff at gyms should always be happy to help guide you.

I have given a goal for the number of reps here, which you'd want to be hitting on the first set. Don't worry if you can't initially sustain that number for the remaining sets; that will come in time as you get stronger. f you'd like to see these and other exercises in action, go to my website (www.theomegaarmy.com/workout-videos).

Push, Pull, Legs

All of these exercises should be done using resistance, either using a barbell or a dumbbell.

	EXERCISE	***REPS***	***SETS***
Day 1: Push	Flat bench press	12	3
	Standing shoulder press	12	3
	Incline bench press	12	3
	Cable flys (high pulley)	12	3
	Tricep extensions	12	3

Day 2: Pull	Pull-ups (assisted or free)	12	3
	Bent-over row	12	3
	Lateral pulldown	12	3
	Upright row	12	3
	Bicep curls	12	3
Day 3: Legs	Back squat	12	3
	Romanian deadlifts	12	3
	Weighted bridge	12	3
	Leg extension	12	3
	Leg curl machine	12	3
	Calf raise machine	12	3

Intermediate Level 2 Workout

If by now you have caught the bodybuilding bug, this is where shit gets real. With this phase, you will be seriously tearing up and rebuilding those fibres. Aim to do these five sessions over the course of a week to see maximum results. You'll move to this level when you feel confident enough to start using free weights for at least half your workouts.

The Bro Split

	EXERCISE	REPS	SETS
Day 1: Chest	Barbell bench press	10	4
	Incline bench press	10	4
	Incline dumbbell flys	10	4
	Close grip bench press	10	4
	Tricep dips (assisted or weighted)	10	4
	Tricep pushdowns	12	3
Day 2: Legs (quad dominant)	Barbell back squats	10	4
	Barbell split squats	10	4
	Leg press machine	10	4
	Walking lunges (on both sides)	10	4
	Leg extension machine	10	4
Day 3: Back	Pull-ups (assisted or weighted)	10	4
	Barbell bent-over rows	10	4
	Lateral pulldowns	10	4
	Rear delt fly	10	4
	Single arm row	10	4
	Barbell bicep curls	10	4
Day 4: Legs (posterior dominant)	Deadlifts	10	3
	Glute bridge	10	4
	Romanian deadlifts	10	4
	Leg machine curls	10	4
	Calf raise machine	10	5

Day 5: Shoulders	Standing overhead press	10	4
	Barbell shrugs	10	4
	Lateral raises	10	4
	Upright row	10	4
	Front raise	10	4

Advanced Level 1

This is a serious bro-split workout, targeting different parts of the body each session, for next-level bodybuilding.

Day 1: Chest

EXERCISE	***REPS***	***SETS***	***%@1RM***
Flat bench press	12	4	60
Incline dumbbell bench press	10	4	60
Dumbbell hex press	10	4	60
Dumbbell flys	10	4	60
Chest pullover	10	4	60
Tricep pushdowns	AMRAP	4	60
Tricep kickbacks (both arms)	AMRAP	3	40

Day 2: Anterior legs (quad-dominant)

EXERCISE	REPS	SETS	%@1RM
Barbell squats	12	4	60
Bulgarian split squats	10	4	60
Leg press machine (with feet close together)	10	4	60
Leg press machine (with feet wide apart) SS	10	4	60
Walking lunges (on both sides)	12	4	45
Leg extension machine	AMRAP	4	60

Day 3: Back

EXERCISE	REPS	SETS	%@1RM
Pull-ups (any grip)	12	4	60
Barbell bent-over row	12	4	60
Reverse pull-up (using body weight)	12	4	60
Wide grip lateral pulldown	12	3	60
Close grip lat pulldown	12	3	60
Single arm rolls	10	4	60
Straight arm pulldown	12	4	60
Standing barbell bicep curls	12	3	50
Concentration curls	12	3	50

Day 4: Posterior legs (hamstring-dominant)

EXERCISE	***REPS***	***SETS***	***%@1RM***
Deadlifts	10	4	60
Weighted bridge	10	4	60
Romanian deadlifts	10	4	60
Nordic curls	10	4	60
Good mornings	10	4	60
Leg curls	10	4	60
Calf raise	12	4	60

Day 5: Shoulders

EXERCISE	***REPS***	***SETS***	***%@1RM***
Standing barbell overhead press	10	4	60
Seated dumbbell shoulder press	10	4	60
Barbell shrugs	10	4	60
Lateral raise	10	4	60
Upright row	10	4	60
Barbell front raise	12	4	60

Advanced Level 2 Workout

This Push, Pull, Legs is all about intensity, as it hits one main muscle group each day. It takes me three to four days to recover from a session like this, and it's the type of workout I feel my body responds to best in terms of making gains.

Day 1: Push (1)

EXERCISE	***REPS***	***SETS***	***%@1RM***
Flat barbell bench press	12	4	60
Seated dumbbell shoulder press	12	4	60
Flat dumbbell flys	12	4	60
Arnold press	12	4	60
Flat dumbbell hex press	12	4	60
Tricep extensions	12	4	60

Day 2: Pull (1)

EXERCISE	***REPS***	***SETS***	***%@1RM***
Bent-over row	12	4	60
Shoulder shrugs	12	4	60
Upright row	12	4	60
Rear delt flys	12	4	60
Front raise	12	4	60
Barbell bicep curls	12	4	60

Day 3: Anterior legs (quad-dominant)

EXERCISE	REPS	SETS	%@1RM
Barbell squats	12	4	60
Bulgarian split squats	10	4	60
Leg press machine (with feet close together)	10	4	60
Leg press machine (with feet wide apart) SS	10	4	60
Walking lunges (on both sides)	12	4	45
Leg extension machine	AMRAP	4	60

Day 4: Push (2)

EXERCISE	REPS	SETS	%@1RM
Standing overhead press	10	4	60
Incline dumbbell chest press	10	4	60
Incline dumbbell flys	10	4	60
Chest pullovers	10	4	60
JM press	10	4	60
Tricep dips	10	4	60

Day 5: Pull (2)

EXERCISE	REPS	SETS	%@1RM
Pull-ups	10	4	60
Wide grip lat pulldowns	10	4	60
Lateral raise	10	4	60
Straight arm pulldown	10	4	60
Single arm dumbbell row	10	4	60
Concentration curls	10	4	60

Day 6: Posterior legs (hamstring-dominant)

EXERCISE	REPS	SETS	%@1RM
Deadlifts	10	4	60
Weighted bridge	10	4	60
Romanian deadlifts	10	4	60
Nordic curls	10	4	60
Good mornings	10	4	60
Leg curls	10	4	60
Calf raise	12	4	60

BODYBUILDING

What bodybuilding delivers: A shredded aesthetic, with a strong upper and lower body.

Why it works: It builds strength by first breaking down the muscle and replenishing protein.

Physique: Chiselled, visibly muscular. Throw away the scales, this will also be about noticing visual changes to your body shape, so take a 'before' picture and another picture each week as your training progresses.

Pros: You will get bigger and become stronger as you recruit more muscle fibres. Your body shape will change to a solid frame, looking aesthetically pleasing in the classic sense.

Cons: Potential injury to the body due to incorrect positioning. For some it can descend into 'ego lifting', whereby you're lifting beyond your ability or without paying proper attention to technique.

Equipment: Lifting belt; weighted belts for pull-ups and dips; three lifting straps to aid grip so you can hold heavier weights – figure of eight strap, standard strap, wrist straps to support wrist joints during heavy lift; knee sleeves for joint protection, warmth and stability; knee wraps (to improve knee safety during heavy squatting; these also give a little bounce). See page 239 for more info.

POWERLIFTING

This section is for anyone passionate about taking strength to the next level. If that isn't a priority for you, you could skirt over this to the next section of the book, otherwise you'll risk becoming as frazzled reading this as I've been writing it.

Newton, Einstein and Turing – if weightlifting had been their thing (and I like to think it might have), powerlifting would have been their strand. This is where the boffins hang out, the muscle geeks who want to train smart and who enjoy training sums and calculations. Don't let that put you off, though; if doing a spot of physics isn't your idea of a party, I have put together some plans for you to help you get your head around it.

A form of strength training, the goal in this sport is to get stronger by moving the heaviest weights you can, doing three main lifts: the squat, bench press and deadlift. Powerlifting has become an increasingly popular training component of other sports as it's so effective at bringing overall strength and power to the body. It's the great love of my life – it goes: sleep, Guinness, my family, and powerlifting right up on top. It has a popular competition aspect, but if the podium doesn't appeal to you (and it doesn't to me), it's still a cracking workout to do, competing against yourself to break your own records, to gradually improve your strength and lifting efficiency. I'm always thinking about the next progression, with numbers whirling round my mind relating to what I'll be lifting this week and how they differ from the week before. It's the only thing that motivates me to go to gym – seeing myself getting stronger and lifting heavier weights.

When you fall in love with powerlifting – and be careful, because you might – you'll become obsessed with the power of the body and the incredible things it can achieve. If you're a novice, you'll learn more about the body in a few months of powerlifting than years practising most other forms of strength training.

I first came across powerlifting during rugby training (where it was used to determine our level of strength and what needed developing), when legendary strength coach, and currently the strongest man in the UK, Adam Bishop was working with the team I played for. Then, after years of mainly focusing on bodybuilding (which is a good gateway for this discipline), I branched out into powerlifting and it's totally changed how I approach fitness. I call myself a power-builder, because I combine bodybuilding with powerlifting, synching both approaches so that one complements the other, on a twelve-week cycle. Bodybuilding focuses more on muscle growth. The larger the muscle, the more contractile force that's produced, so a bodybuilder might look like a unit, but powerlifters can often lift more weight. This strand of weightlifting incorporates a much more cognitive approach than just bashing out rep after rep, which I'd previously done. It's not one of those sports where you'll be sweating buckets after a workout; there are more subtle things happening behind the scenes, both physically as you build more muscle and mentally as you tap into your central nervous system.

Full disclosure: my main incentive for starting to power-lift a few years back was ego-based. I loved smashing heavy weights and I wanted the world to know about it, so I'd post my max on Insta with the aim of getting likes. And it worked. People really loved seeing the mad shit I was lifting and, as tragic as the case may be, I lapped it up. So, I went to town – *lift, lift, lift, boom, boom, boom* – with not much time for rest and recovery, which is a vital component of powerlifting. I had moved from doing six days a week of bodybuilding to applying the same no-pain-no-gain mentality to powerlifting. Disaster. After some initial impressive gains, I fucked my system; I was totally exhausted and fatigued, and it caused a burnout I'm still recovering from. What went wrong? Well, powerlifting relies heavily on mental energy, recruiting motor units through central-nervous-system stimulus. Whereas bodybuilding draws on high-rep metabolic stress, powerlifting is more about mechanical tension (see page 201 for a recap). Going max-capacity at every session, and hitting the gym too many times a week, meant my CNS couldn't recover between sessions. I hadn't learned to work in harmony with it; instead I was essentially telling it to go fuck itself while I ignored any warning signs of fatigue, thinking that rest could hold me back on the progress I was determined to make. I convinced myself I was tougher than that. I wasn't, and it caught up with me. Eighteen months later, I'm still managing knee and back pain which could have been avoided if I'd listened to my body and set aside my pride.

I'm behaving myself these days, with any notions above my station firmly in check. That doesn't mean I need to curb my ambition; it just means I need to be more sensible in achieving my goals – a slow-and-steady-wins-the-race approach that means I gradually get stronger. In practice, this will allow me to continue powerlifting safely well into my forties and fifties if I want to.

It's helpful to have done strength training before starting, but it's not essential. Even if you're brand new and totally unfit, with some weight to shed (in fact, if you are overweight, it likely means you have natural strength and are forceful), jump in, my friend, and you won't look back. You'll probably do more volume at the start in order to get your technique right for the three main lifts.

And so to the importance of form and technique, both of which are vital to get right, to lift as ergonomically as possible as well as to avoid injury (take it from me, you do not want to do a deadlift without proper technique). If possible, I'd recommend getting a coach to guide you through a twelve-week macro-cycle or a micro-cycle (more info on this coming up), so that you can learn basic form. This is because PTs on most commercial gym floors won't have the expertise to advise on technique. If hiring a powerlifting coach isn't an option, don't worry, because there are lots of good resources online. If you really catch powerlifting fever and decide to join a lifters' gym (which will have more specialist equipment, and membership costs are relatively low), you'll probably find that fellow lifters there will be pretty vocal when observing your moves and telling you what's what! There's often good banter as well as serious know-how to learn from. These are my people.

Strongman/woman

This is a sport where people train using specialist equipment in Strongman/woman gyms. Think of a spartan warrior god/goddess – their closest modern-day relative will be a Strongman/woman – 6ft 5ins and 140kg of sheer power. There's some crossover between powerlifting and Strongman/woman, with undulating periodisation involved in both types of training, and some people dabble in both sports.

Strongmen and women all share a goal of being the strongest person in the world, and they are completely dedicated to working towards that. A rigorous training programme becomes engrained in your lifestyle if you're serious about it. You'll be at the gym every day, sometimes eating up to 10,000 calories a day (expensive and not easy on the digestion!). These athletes really take strength to a new level.

> 'Being the strongest human on the planet is the ultimate goal. I value strength over any other component of fitness. The best thing is there's no upper limit – how strong I get is up to me and me alone, how much I put into the process and how much I want to succeed.'
>
> ADAM BISHOP, BRITAIN'S STRONGEST MAN 2020

Powerlifting maths 101

Powerlifting = intensity × maximal effort × specificity

Powerlifters speak a whole other language, and this is where your formulas for programming come in, which I explain here. At first glance, it might appear mind-boggling, but it'll quickly make sense once you start following the workout plan.

Your powerlifting dictionary

Programming: This is your powerlifting routine – the strategic weekly or monthly schedule that you follow, with a view to improving your rep max and overall strength. Good programming breaks down mental barriers, because when you have a great plan in front of you, you know that there's method to the madness and you will get gains. Part of the reason I backtracked with my powerlifting progress was because of shit programming. I had made linear gains, but when linear progression was no longer enough for me to progress, I knew I'd shut down my CNS, not helped by omitting de-load days (see below).

Specificity: The training programme tailored especially to your needs, depending on the outcome you want to achieve, so the training you do should all focus on improving your three main lifts.

Rep max (RM): It's all about heavy weights rather than reps as you load the movements.

Macro-cycles: A bigger plan, often 12 weeks, made up of micro-cycles.

Micro-cycles: 1–4 weeks of a programme, forming part of a macro-cycle.

The law of accommodation: As with any type of exercise you do, when your body gets used to a stimulus (i.e. a particular type of training), its effect on the body decreases. To avoid accommodation, you need to vary your exercise regime.

Accessory/assistance work: After your main lifts, these are the training exercises you do towards the end of the workout. It's a way of bodybuilding to achieve bigger muscles, building on the training you've done in the session (depending on your upper-/lower-body focus that day). They tend to be variances of the big lifts but less strenuous on the body because of the lower intensity and volume used.

Competition max (100%) and a gym max (90%): When training, you never work to a 100% effort because you would overdo it; you save that for if you're competing or on the occasion you want to test your total strength. Think of it like a long-distance runner never doing the full 26.1 miles before marathon day.

De-load periods: You need to give your body a chance to recover after high-intensity training. A de-load will typically last a week and, depending on your programming, it tends to mean reducing volume by about 50% (e.g. if you had been bench-pressing 100kg for 10 reps, you'd reduce it to 100kg for 5 reps during the de-load phase), or even doing no training whatsoever. Make sure you don't decrease the weight; it's the volume that you reduce. This is an absolutely essential component of powerlifting once you reach intermediate level and beyond. The strain for an elite lifter is much more on the mind than the body. If rest isn't adhered to, this will slow, or even reverse, your progress and cause CNS fatigue, burnout and injury.

If you are a beginner, don't worry just yet about scheduling de-load weeks because you're not yet lifting the loads required to put stress on the CNS – you'll still be at the stage of switching on your receptors. Until you begin to plateau, that won't be necessary. You'll know when you stop making lifting gains of 2.5–5kg every week that you're coming into an intermediate stage, and you'll need to start factoring them in.

Fatigue debt (high and low): This is the energy debt which comes as a result of training. A **high** debt is where you give it everything you've got. This is a short-term strategy that you might use if you're competing and have a tournament coming up. During the weeks before, you'd go all out in training to build strength and force. In your twenties, high fatigue is easier, but as you get older, it takes its toll on your body. I got really strong really fast doing high fatigue, but it led to burnout. However, training with a **low** fatigue debt (such as the linear-progression method) is a slower, steadier way to get gradually stronger (you should see a 1% increase in strength every 12 weeks). It tends to result in fewer injuries and is a more sustainable, long-term way of training.

Recovery: Rest in its different forms is integral to powerlifting. Firstly, the benefits of a good night's sleep (see page 285) are among of the greatest gifts you can give a powerlifter. Then there's de-loading, which you now know about, and finally, to facilitate stimulus recovery and adaption, you'll be resting different parts of the body and muscle groups by alternating your training. When you're doing lower or dynamic effort lower and upper (for example, if you're following the conjugate method, see page 245), you need to take off at least a day or two afterwards because your CNS will be pretty tired. This kind of mechanical tension has a similar effect on the body as the fight-or-flight response (see page 70). I've told you already about how I was addicted to the pump (metabolic stress) and a total gobshite for not resting. So, learn from my mistakes!

Ramping weights: This is a gradual loading of weights in a session, working your way up to heavier ones for your top set. So, your first set might be 100kg × 5 reps, then 120 × 5, 140 × 5 and then to 160 × 5 – keep going for a bigger amount.

Myofibrillar hypertrophy: This is the reason that powerlifters tend to look less stacked than bodybuilders, even when they are stronger. It comes about by using heavier weights with a lower number of repetitions. This makes the muscle stronger because the heavier the weight you lift, the more micro-tears in the muscle, which increases the myofibril size – so your strength will increase but you may not see a big difference in the size of the muscle. Meanwhile, bodybuilding draws on sarcoplasmic hypertrophy, which increases the muscles' glycogen storage, making them swell but having less of an impact on their actual strength.

Sensory input to motor output: Signals carried from the brain to the rest of the body, which in the context of weightlifting tell your body to pick up a weight and how much force will be needed to do so. You can increase your capacity to receive more sensory input, meaning your body will become more efficient at lifting effectively. As you develop this CNS adaptation during your progress as a powerlifter, by doing deliberate reprogramming exercises like big compound lifts, your body will become quicker and more powerful.

Stimulus Recover Adaption (SRA) curve: During training our bodies respond to stimuli, and what makes them stronger is their ability to adapt. The curve is used to understand the phases your body goes through while training and recovering.

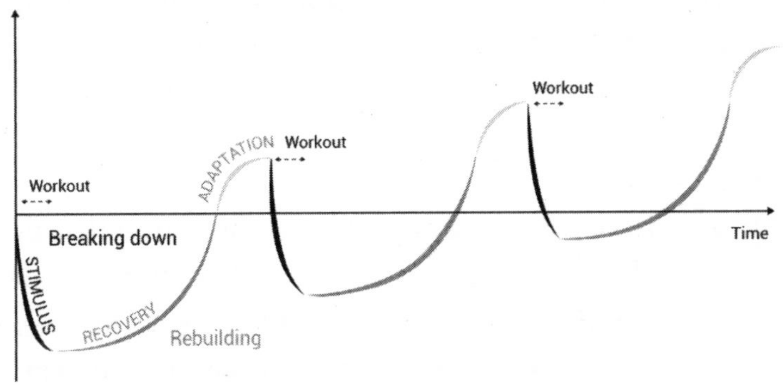

SRA curve

Bands and chains: Some training systems use these to accommodate extra resistance, adding a new stimulus. The tension in the bands provides extra kinetic energy while the chains give extra weight in different areas of your lift – as they come up off the floor, more weight goes onto the bar. If you are in the bottom of a deadlift and you start lifting the bar, while you might only have 20kg of chains on there, as you lift the bar up towards the top of the lift, it'll have become much heavier, feeling more like an extra 60kg.

RPE scale: This is a way to assess the difficulty range of what you're doing so that you know how much further to push yourself in a training session. From 0 to 10 – 0 being easy and 10 being your max. It's a bit like the scale doctors use to assess pain – and you should be in pain during your powerlifting session! If your RPE is at a 7, it means you can do three more reps. It's another way of helping you tune into how your body is feeling, and this will become easier and easier the more you train and get to know your body. There's also the 6 to 20 method (also called the Borg Scale), but the RPE scale is easier to follow and to me makes a lot more sense (6 to 20 as an assessment feels random).

Technique

Using your breath and bracing

If you're bodybuilding, you might be able to get away with not focusing too much on the breath, but when you come to lift the really heavy stuff, like when you're powerlifting, you've got to be more aware. In the past, when I was less experienced, I've thrown out my back and damaged my SI joints (the sacroiliac joints, which connect the spine to the pelvis) from not bracing while doing big lifts. If you've watched events such as Strongman/woman competitions, you may have seen lifters move the most enormous weights, and as soon as the lift is over, they'll collapse to the ground, sometimes passing out or with nosebleeds. It's quite the advert for the sport! One of the reasons they might keel over after giving the lift their absolute all is because they're lightheaded, having held their breath.

A weight belt will help protect your back, but you must also learn to harness your breath and brace. Proper breathing techniques and good form go hand in hand. Bracing will help you engage your core, making that whole area rigid, where it's usually softer.

So, when I go into a deadlift or squat, I breathe into my belly, expanding it as far as it'll go and holding it there while I do a rep (this will take around five seconds), after which I release through my nose or mouth.

If you're trying to get the hang of bracing, practise with a lighter weight as it'll be easier to finesse your technique.

Equipment

If you're doing equipped, rather than raw, powerlifting, here's some of the kit to consider, all of which is approved for use by the International Powerlifting Federation. Some of these contraptions are for safety while you lift, whereas others are more performance-enhancers. People feel differently about the use of accessories which during a competition will boost your personal best, and there's something about them that doesn't quite sit right with me. I feel they're questionable because they unnaturally enhance your lifts, and that doesn't seem fair. You might see people wearing these in the gym, but they're primarily used in competitions.

Bench shirt: This super-tight shirt gives you a spring when you do a bench press; it creates extra friction and gives a bounce to lifts.

Squat suit: These suits are so tight you have to have someone to help squeeze you into them, so here's hoping you have some friends nearby. They give extra support when lifting very heavy weights and help maintain good alignment.

Deadlift suit: Similar to the above, they're so compact that you spring off the top or off the bottom of your deadlift, helping you bounce up.

Knee wraps: These provide extra stability to the knee joints and give a 10% boost, providing you with a little spring out of the bottom of your squats.

Wrist straps: I use these to help protect my wrists, keeping them nice and solid during any pressing motions, but people also use them while they're squatting.

Knee sleeves: These keep the knees warm and limber; they're not as effective as knee wraps with helping you to push, but they can make you feel safer when wearing them.

Weightlifting belts: These create intra-abdominal pressure and everyone should use them to protect the back from injury when lifting heavy weights.

Singlets: These are form-fitting suits worn at weightlifting events, tightening the body into position in preparation for a lift.

Single-ply and multi-ply shirts: These tight tops give you a spring when you bench press. The single-ply shirts are made from a thinner layer of material whereas the multi-ply is thicker (and even tighter).

Squat shoes: Some people choose lifting shoes that drive more pressure towards the quads, while others prefer to stick their bums out and break parallel before they stand back up, so they wear flat shoes or ones with a small heel, allowing them to sit more upright in a squat.

Deadlifting shoes: These are flat shoes or slippers which help to keep you as low and as close to the floor as you can be when you're doing a deadlift. Trainers tend to have a raised sole, putting you at a deficit, whereas flat lifting shoes will allow you to drop down around an inch.

Chalk: This is applied to your hands to help you grip the bar. It can also be applied on your back, quads and shins when doing different exercises to help avoid tearing the skin while moving the weight. Can be used liberally.

Ammonia: Imagine a Victorian lady's smelling salts – this is effectively the same thing. It might be used before some reps as a little pick-me-up to help bring focus.

The main training programmes

Just as there's more than one way to skin a cat, there are different approaches to powerlifting training, and here I'll talk you through some of the ones I rate the most that cater for different levels of experience and aptitude. Something they all have in common is that they all aim to get you stronger by frequently changing up the stimulus and, in turn, recruiting more motor units. Powerlifting training sessions will move between quick-speed days, high-strain days, max-effort days, dynamic days, and the rep method (based on bodybuilding). The theory behind each method is that you get stronger while doing accessory work (remember, these are the variations of the main lift which complement your training). Some people stick to one method in their training while others mix them up. As you progress, you'll start to home in on what works for you and what you enjoy.

As always, before trying any new movements, ask a training expert at the gym to talk you through specific lifts and then to observe you, making sure you're in the optimal position each time, keeping safety paramount.

The linear-progression method

For the advanced, this is all about the magic 1% – becoming 1% stronger after completing a twelve-week cycle. It's a great place for novices to start as it builds solid foundations, and for intermediates to continue to progress, beginning with a four-week micro-cycle involving intense training followed by a de-load week (remember de-loading is only required once you progress past beginner level and start plateauing), where you'll be allowing your body to recover from the strain of the previous weeks. During the first three weeks, you'll be ramping weights, increasing the weights in small increments each week. You'd then de-load during Week 4, before the cycle continues again on Week 5, progressing from where you left off on week three. Here's an example of what a twelve-week linear progression macro-cycle might entail, focusing on the squat, bench press, deadlift and overhead press (one each day, over four days). (The overhead press isn't always embraced by powerlifters as it's not one of the three key moves, but I like it because it works the triceps and can help your personal best.) The de-load weeks are factored in, where you take it easy, keeping the weight but decreasing the sets and reps. You'll see that as you get stronger, the emphasis is on lifting heavier weights but for a lower number of repetitions.

Example of a linear progression macro-cycle:

MICRO-CYCLE 1	WEEK	VOLUME	REPS	SETS
	1	50kg	8	4
	2	55kg	8	4
	3	60kg	8	4
	4	65kg	8	4
De-load (if at intermediate level)				

MICRO-CYCLE 2	WEEK	VOLUME	REPS	SETS
	5	75kg	5	5
	6	80kg	5	5
	7	85kg	5	5
	8	90kg	5	5
De-load (if at intermediate level)				

MICRO-CYCLE 3	WEEK	VOLUME	REPS	SETS
	9	100kg	3	10
	10	105kg	3	10
	11	110kg	3	10
	12	115kg	3	10
De-load (if at intermediate level)				

After this macro-cycle, you'd then begin a new one, starting Week 1 lifting 55–65kg for four sets of eight reps. For the less mentally-tough option, start at 55kg, but if you're really feeling that you could have done more, go for 65kg. This is why I love this slowly-slowly approach: it lays a solid foundation for growth that can be easily measured.

If you are new to powerlifting, you'll quickly notice your strength improving and you'll have a new 1RM (see page 208) every week as you measure the gains from the previous week's work. Seeing your numbers written down in black and white (or in the notes section of your phone, as the case may be!) is what will drive your competitive edge; you'll become hooked on beating yourself. As you progress to intermediate level, you should have a new 1RM. Remember, though, you never do your max effort during training.

The Texas method

This is a solid way to programme, for beginners and intermediates, which I have used for the intermediate workout coming up. It follows a three-day-a-week timetable (so it makes it easier to slot in for the time-poor, provided you use the three sessions at the gym effectively) that divides each workout between high-volume lifts, recovery and high intensity for the major lifts. It utilises wave loading, an approach to training that builds strength by mixing up the intensity of sets, going from high to medium then to low before a rest. It's a volume method, so on the volume day you'll be doing 5 × 5 on squats, then an upper-body lift and a lower-body variant pull exercise. On the 'rest' day (in fairness, it's more of a 'lighter' day than a rest day), you'll be doing 80% of your volume day. On the high-intensity day, you'll do three major lifts where you try to achieve a new personal-record (PR) 5 rep max (until your body reaches a plateau). The constant, rapid changes stimulate adaption as the muscles are shocked into working at different paces. The recovery periods are strategically factored in and it's during these times that muscles grow, something that's called 'active rest'. Getting the nutrition you need as well as decent sleep is super-important with this method.

The 5-3-1 method

This is a straightforward and steady way to programme, based around the four main lifts (squat, bench press, deadlift and overhead), focusing on one of them in each session. With this method, you only ever work off your training max, never your 'real' or competition max.

So the 5-3-1 element would come in this way:

Week 1:	65% × 5 reps
	75% × 5 reps
	85% × 5+ (AMRAP)
Week 2:	70% × 3 reps
	80% × 3 reps
	90% × 3+ (AMRAP)
Week 3:	75% × 5 reps
	85% × 3 reps
	95% × 1
Week 4:	De-load

The conjugate method

I couldn't write about powerlifting without including this legendary training approach. It's not the one I include in the actual workout plan, but it has had so much influence on powerlifting that I'm giving it a shout-out here.

Also known as the Westside Barbell method, named for the American gym where it was created in the 1980s after they started studying Russian strength training manuals (Russia and other Eastern bloc countries were ahead of the game on harnessing strategies for how to build strength). It's become a popular programme followed by intermediate and elite lifters, and has been proven to get results. Again, it splits the training sessions into upper body (overhead press, bench press) and lower body (squat and deadlift). One of the mantras in weightlifting is that there are a thousand ways to perform a certain lift, and this type of training is all about doing those variations, the aim being that variations in the movement, even small ones, will shock your CNS, forcing it to recruit more muscle fibres. So, you'll do your squats during one training session a slightly different way to the ones you did last time.

Back in the day, the guys at Westside gym were working out to the full at every session, putting in all their effort and commitment, but found they were actually losing strength. They figured out that the body simply can't max out at every workout and the way to get stronger would happen by alternating training between days that focused on strength (maximal effort days) and those all about speed (dynamic effort days). Here, the various components of strength can all be developed alongside each other, rather than, for example, strength being built up to the detriment of speed. Max effort days are about how you feel, and you need to listen to yourself so that you don't overdo it. For example, my max deadlift is 330kg – if I was doing paused deadlifts, I'd start at 100kg and increase the weight slowly, going to 140kg, then to 180kg, then to 220kg and then to 250kg. My max effort that day might be 280kg for eight reps. Then my next exercises will be 80% of my top set that day (280kg) – so five sets of paused deadlifts at 235kg.

Undulating periodisation

This is the top programme used by the most elite powerlifters in the world. It works by mixing up the stimulus, alternating between low volume with higher intensity and high volume with lower intensity, making the body very responsive to progress. Unlike the linear-progression method, where the volume and intensity are increased at a gradual level, here the phases of higher and lower volume are alternated, as are the levels of intensity. Essentially, you train one area of the body hard before moving onto the next, and it also works on the CNS to recruit motor units, but not to over-tire it.

Some lifters also find it to be effective at staving off injury, because you only train one system for a short time before moving to the next. The lifters who programme in this way are at the peak of what they can do. There's no point in doing this until you're at an advanced level as your body will still make more gains with the other methods I've covered. The advanced powerlifting plan I've put together is undulating periodisation, which you can implement once you've reached the peak of your powers.

And – *breathe.* Your powerlifting lesson is over. Hard on the brain, wasn't it?

Beginner's workout

Linear progression

This plan gives a four-day schedule for two weeks, and you should take a day off in between each workout. Keep adding weight until you start to hit a plateau at 2.5kg, after which you can start other programmes to keep you progressing. It should be done at 90% of your 5 rep max and you can add plus-sets at the end of the week (on the last set, instead of 5 reps, you do as many as possible). If you need guidance on any of the movements here, make sure you ask a trainer at the gym or have a look at www.theomegaarmy.com/workout-videos.

WEEK 1

DAY 1

EXERCISE	***REPS***	***SETS***	***%***	***SET 1***	***SET 2***	***SET 3***	***SET 4***	***SET 5***
Squat	5	3	60					
Bench	5	3	60					
Deadlift	5	1	60					

DAY 2

EXERCISE	***REPS***	***SETS***	***%***	***SET 1***	***SET 2***	***SET 3***	***SET 4***	***SET 5***
Squat	5	3	60					
Overhead press	5	3	60					
Deadlift	5	1	60					

WEEK 2

DAY 1

EXERCISE	REPS	SETS	%	SET 1	SET 2	SET 3	SET 4	SET 5
Squat	5	5	60					
Bench	5	5	60					
Deadlift	5	1	60					

DAY 2

EXERCISE	REPS	SETS	%	SET 1	SET 2	SET 3	SET 4	SET 5
Squat	5	5	60					
Overhead press	5	5	60					
Weighted pull-up	5	3	60					

Intermediate workout

Texas method

WEEK 1

DAY 1 VOLUME (YOU CAN ADD PLUS-SETS ON THE LAST SETS)

EXERCISE	***REPS***	***SETS***	***5RM%***
Squat	5	5	90
Overhead press	5	5	90
Heavy pulldown	5	5	90

DAY 2 RECOVERY

EXERCISE	***REPS***	***SETS***	***%***
Squat	5	3	80
Overhead press	5	3	80
Heavy pulldown	5	3	80

DAY 3 INTENSITY (INCREASE WEIGHTS UP TO THE TOP SET)

EXERCISE	***REPS***	***SETS***	***%***
Squat	5	1	Max
Bench	5	1	Max
Deadlift	5	1	Max

Advanced workout

Undulating periodisation

WEEK 1

DAY 1

EXERCISE	***REPS***	***SETS***	***%***	***SET 1***	***SET 2***	***SET 3***	***SET 4***	***SET 5***
High bar squat	8	3	65					
Bulgarian split squat	10	3	70 of top set					
Leg press	10	3	55					
Leg extension	10	3	55					
Glute ham raise	10	3	50					

DAY 2

EXERCISE	***REPS***	***SETS***	***%***	***SET 1***	***SET 2***	***SET 3***	***SET 4***	***SET 5***
Bench press	5	5	75					
Incline DB press	8	5	80 of top set					
JM press	10	3	55					
Dips	10	3	55					
Tricep extension	10	3	50					

DAY 3

EXERCISE	***REPS***	***SETS***	***%***	***SET 1***	***SET 2***	***SET 3***	***SET 4***	***SET 5***
Deadlift	3	3	85					
Paused deadlift	5	3	80 of top set					
Explosive deadlift	3	6	65					
Barbell rows	10	3	55					
Stiff leg deadlifts	10	3	55					

DAY 4

EXERCISE	***REPS***	***SETS***	***%***	***SET 1***	***SET 2***	***SET 3***	***SET 4***	***SET 5***
Low bar squat	5	5	75					
Front squats	8	5	80 of top set					
Leg press	10	3	55					
Leg extension	10	3	55					

DAY 5

EXERCISE	**REPS**	**SETS**	**%**	**SET 1**	**SET 2**	**SET 3**	**SET 4**	**SET 5**
Bench press	3	3	85					
Incline barbell bench	5	3	80 of top set					
Dumbbell hex press	6	3	65					
DB flys	10	3	55					
Low pulley fly	10	3	55					

DAY 6

EXERCISE	**REPS**	**SETS**	**%**	**SET 1**	**SET 2**	**SET 3**	**SET 4**	**SET 5**
Deadlift	3	3	60					
Paused deadlift	5	3	80 of top set					
Explosive deadlift	3	6	40					
Barbell rows	10	3	57.5					
Stiff leg deadlifts	10	3	57.5					

WEEK 2

DAY 1

EXERCISE	REPS	SETS	%	SET 1	SET 2	SET 3	SET 4	SET 5
High bar squat	3	3	85					
Paused squats	5	3	80 of top set					
Leg press	10	3	57.5					
Leg extension	10	3	57.5					
Glute ham raise	10	3	55					

DAY 2

EXERCISE	REPS	SETS	%	SET 1	SET 2	SET 3	SET 4	SET 5
Bench press	8	3	65					
Incline DB press	10	3	70 of top set					
JM press	10	3	57.5					
Dips	10	3	57.5					
Tricep extension	10	3	57.5					

DAY 3

EXERCISE	***REPS***	***SETS***	***%***	***SET 1***	***SET 2***	***SET 3***	***SET 4***	***SET 5***
Deadlift	8	3	65					
Paused deadlift	5	3	80 of top set					
Explosive deadlift	3	6	55					
Barbell rows	10	3	57.5					
Stiff leg deadlifts	10	3	57.5					

DAY 4

EXERCISE	***REPS***	***SETS***	***%***	***SET 1***	***SET 2***	***SET 3***	***SET 4***	***SET 5***
High bar squat	8	3	70					
Bulgarian split squat	10	3	70 of top set					
Leg press	10	3	57.5					
Leg extension	10	3	57.5					
Glute ham raise	10	3	55					

DAY 5

EXERCISE	*REPS*	*SETS*	*%*	*SET 1*	*SET 2*	*SET 3*	*SET 4*	*SET 5*
Bench press	5	5	77.5					
Incline DB press	8	5	80 of top set					
JM press	10	3	57.5					
Dips	10	3	57.5					
Tricep extension	10	3	55					

DAY 6

EXERCISE	*REPS*	*SETS*	*%*	*SET 1*	*SET 2*	*SET 3*	*SET 4*	*SET 5*
Deadlift	3	3	62.5					
Paused deadlift	5	3	80 of top set					
Explosive dead	3	6	45					
Barbell rows	10	3	60					
Stiff leg deadlifts	10	3	60					

POWERLIFTING

What powerlifting delivers: Strength in your three main lifts – the squat, bench press and deadlift.

Why it works: Varying the stimulus through twelve-week macro-cycles programmes your CNS to recruit more motor units, building strength from there. Depending on the type of training you're doing, you should see weekly gains if rotating cycles.

Physique: Less muscly than a bodybuilder, but still stacked in both the upper and lower body.

Pros: It makes the body stronger – and your arithmetic will improve!

Cons: Can cause CNS burnout if you don't give your body time to recover and there is the potential for injury to muscles, tendons and joints due to incorrect positioning or excess stress.

Equipment: See page 239.

Training frequency: Up to four days a week.

Importance of technique: Always ask an expert at the gym to check your form when you lift, especially when doing the squat, bench press and deadlift.

PART 4

YOUR WHOLE-BODY HEALTH

By this stage, I hope I've convinced you to get your arse in gear and push yourself towards greater fitness goals. But all that will only go so far if the rest of your wellbeing is a shit-show.

And, yep, if you've heard it once in this book, you've heard it a million times: it's time to start seeing yourself as a whole entity, the mind and body operating in tandem, if only because working on the whole picture will hugely improve success. For example, you can do all the lifting you like, but if you're not eating to maximise your workouts, or giving yourself time to recover, you won't see the results.

What might surprise you to know is that you could have been working out for years thinking your exercise of choice was having one impact on your body, when actually it was having quite another.

NUTRITION

I've always given clients a nutrition plan tailored to their specific training regime, including calories to aim for as well as targets for protein intake. There aren't any quick fixes to nutrition; it's about making big-picture choices that support your training and overall health. With this in mind, I never give clients a rigid meal plan to follow, specifying meal times along with what should be eaten on what days. In my opinion, being very fixed and restricting freedom around food choices can cause more anxiety around eating. Plus, some days you'll want to eat a steak, while others you might fancy some salmon for dinner, so just go with the flow. I've often heard from clients who have previously followed a food plan that once the weeks are up, they feel a bit at sea, unclear about the choices they should be making now that they're going it alone. By knowing a bit more about the nutrients your body needs and how you can support it during training, it'll mean you make more considered approaches, keeping in mind your long-term goals.

What we eat (or don't eat) impacts how we look, how we feel in terms of day-to-day wellbeing and energy levels, our performance when we exercise and how quickly our body repairs after physical activity. Our food choices can also impact on our future health, with many common diseases such as type 2 diabetes being exacerbated by an unhealthy diet. Not only can certain conditions be preventable through our lifestyle, they can sometimes also be reversed through a diet and fitness overhaul as the body repairs itself (thanks, body). I know I've used the term food 'choices', but in reality it doesn't always feel that much of a choice, does it? For example, when you're tired or stressed, it's totally understandable that we reach for high-sugar or high-fat foods, just to give us the energy to make it through the day. This turns into a bit of a vicious cycle when you eat lots of dodgy food, because you're exhausted, but in the long run those foods deplete your energy even further and lead to other health issues.

Approaches to nutrition

> 'Diet culture is systematically ruining our ability to reach our fitness goals while enjoying the food we eat. It needs to stop. To find true happiness with food and achieve our fitness goals, diet culture first needs to be removed from the process.'
>
> GRAEME TOMLINSON, THE FITNESS CHEF

If you find it hard to keep up with the latest food fads, getting all in a tizz about what the hell paleo or ketogenic actually mean, then you're in good company. I'm as bemused as anyone else about the rise in diet-mania. In my opinion there seems to be questionable science behind many diets or simply not enough research to comment one way or the other. The recent controversy of skinny jabs as appetite suppressants, advertised by some celebrities (in what seems to me a very irresponsible way), is a case in point of the world gone mad. Not that meal replacements are particularly new, but it's a shame that our quick-fix obsession seems more about punishing yourself than looking after your health. And often these diet 'solutions' are aimed at young women, even girls. My own daughter isn't too far off being a teenager and it annoys me to think of her and her friends being targeted by these absurd, dangerous products.

Whether you are vegan, avoid gluten or fast intermittently, you need to find an approach to eating that makes you feel good and supports your whole-body health, regardless of what glossy magazines are telling you is in food fashion from one month to the next. There's no 'good' food or 'bad' food – it's just food! And provided you have an eye on portion sizes, keeping moderation in mind as well as the energy you are expending, there are no such thing as 'forbidden' foods. You don't need to go all MasterChef, but the ingredients you choose should keep you energised, especially as you'll hopefully be using your diet to sustain an active lifestyle. The way you eat needs to work for you long-term, because radical or extreme diets don't tend to work.

How we eat

I'm not going to start lecturing you about your diet (well, I am a bit), and I won't pretend my life is all quinoa, kale and spirulina (although actually quinoa is a good source of protein so I occasionally dabble!). The reason I'm including info about food is not because I'm a Jamie Oliver in the kitchen (beans on toast is considered gourmet in my house) but, as you might expect, because it really will make a big difference to your overall fitness. There's no point toiling away in the gym or on the pitch only for your diet to undermine your progress.

It's common sense that decent-quality, nourishing foods should make up the bulk of your calories every day. By this I mean a variety of protein-rich meat, fish, dairy or plant-based foods (more on that coming up), wholesome carbohydrates, healthy fats, and plenty of veg and fruit (fresh or frozen are the best options; remember if you're using tins that other ingredients may have been added). These foods contain combinations of macronutrients (protein, fat and carbohydrates) and micronutrients (vitamins and minerals) as well as other goodies like fibre and antioxidants.

That being said, I am partial to the occasional takeout,

and I know that because I work so hard at the gym, this will have zero detrimental impact on my physique or training. I have no hang-ups or guilt around food; my attitude towards it is that by and large it's fuel that gives me energy to train, and most of what I eat is good stuff that, as well as giving me energy, is providing my body with essential nutrients to be healthy and stave off illness as far as possible. So, if I'm eating out or getting in a pizza every so often, then I'll enjoy it, knowing that a balance has been struck. When you cook as many meals as I do in a day, ordering in is a joy. But before you speed-dial Domino's I need to stress there that I work on the basis of a calorie surplus, and many of you reading this will not be. I need to hit around 4,000 calories a day, so an occasional takeaway pizza, which is around 1,000 calories, is going to fit fine within my overall target.

Here's a typical day for me – and remember, this is almost twice as much as the recommended daily intake for someone less active. The first thing I do when I wake is make a shake, adding a 25g scoop of protein. About an hour and a half later I'll have a big bowl of porridge with berries or cereal. Mid-morning I'll whip up a four-egg omelette and eat that with four slices of buttered toast. After hitting the gym, I'll drink another protein shake, this time made with two scoops of protein. Lunch will be a steak or salmon fillet along with some brown rice and veg. Dinner might be a big bowl of pasta served with another hit of protein, like chicken, and some salad or cooked veg on the side. If I'm hungry again later in the evening (and I usually am!) I'll snack on nuts, protein bars and fruit, or have a bowl of cereal. I like a glass of red wine in the evening too – medicinal, obviously (my body is a temple . . .). The intensity of my training means my muscles need this high number of calories, but if I was eating all this and not burning it off, I would be seriously overweight and not healthy.

There have been times when I've been injured that I have had to reduce my training and as a result I might put on weight. I never worry about this, as I know I will easily lose it when I return to sport. It's not realistic to think you will hit your dream weight or physique and then stay like that for the rest of your life; it's just not going to happen, as life will get in the way (and so it should). A certain amount of fluctuation is totally normal and natural.

My opinion is that if most of the food we eat is nourishing, with a small proportion of it less so, and provided we are active, it is very unlikely to affect our performance. When you are more in tune with your body and your eating habits, this will become more instinctive. And the point is that when you are exercising effectively, you can be much more free in your food choices.

Calories and energy balance

The amount of energy in our food and drink is measured in units called calories. Very simply, energy balance is just the number of calories you consume through food versus the calories you expend through moving as well as the rate at which your body burns calories when you are at rest (called the basic metabolic rate). This is where the body does its millions of automated functions to keep you alive, e.g. pumping blood around the body and keeping that ticker going. If you burn more calories than you eat, you will lose weight, and if you eat more than you burn, then the reverse is true. If you are restricting calories, it makes sense to choose calories from wholesome foods that are filling and will boost energy. If you 'spend' your calories on junk food, it won't sustain you for as long and might lead to a blood sugar imbalance, where it initially gives you a burst of energy but then makes you feel shit.

Calories are listed on packets of food and drinks, and for fresh, unpackaged ingredients there are many apps that will tell you the calories they contain. What you eat will have different effects on your body, based on the nutrients it contains (more of that coming up). If you are trying to monitor the number of calories consumed in a day, it's a good idea to keep track using an app. Log your calories weekly, though, rather than daily, and it'll mean you can then use any surplus to do with what you will – a little of what you fancy does you good, after all. If you're filthy rich and don't enjoy cooking, or if you just want to take the thinking out of it all, you might consider using one of those home-delivery services that prepares meals tailored to your nutritional/calorific needs. Sorry, kids, there goes the college fund . . .

Calorie deficit

This just means reducing your calories and/or increasing your energy expenditure in order to lose fat. I get bombarded with questions about how to lose body fat and get more lean (often from those who say in the same breath that they want to get a #hotbod in order to appeal to a certain lady or gent – who am I to get in the way of true lust?). I could win an award for stating the bleedin' obvious here but I give the age-old advice to start with: eating less, moving more.

I never recommend a drastic cut in daily calories when

combined with training, even for someone who has a good bit of weight to lose. A maximum 15% decrease in your daily calorie intake is a much more sustainable and consistent approach; any more than that and it's hard to stick at it, unless you have a military mindset. Cutting calories, combined with whatever exercise appeals, will change your body shape. Simple as that. And if it's your abs you want to say hello to in the mirror, losing fat will be just as, if not more, effective for gaining definition there.

For safe ways to create a deficit:

- Watch your portion sizes, especially if you're eating out – restaurant serving sizes are often double the recommended amount.
- Make sure you hit your protein goals, eating it at every meal – not just so that you build or maintain muscle mass but also because it's filling.
- Make substitutes: foods like wholegrain pasta and bread tend to be lower in calories than their white friends.
- Keep hydrated: sometimes the body mistakes hunger for thirst.
- Make it easier for yourself by keeping your kitchen packed with healthy, lower-calorie nosh, especially if you're the snacking type.

The body is skilled at adapting and you'll probably find that while the first days of a calorie deficit can be filled with hangry rage, you'll quickly get used to eating a little less (remember, no more than 15%) and you'll be satisfied with fewer calories.

Calorie surplus

Depending on how much exercise you're doing, as well as your wider fitness and health goals, you may find yourself increasing your daily calories. You'll need to do this if you're wanting to build muscle because it's not possible to do that in a deficit. This allows muscles to remain in anabolism i.e. the process that strengthens or maintains your muscle mass. Again, I'd always recommend a modest increase as you progress, beginning with no more than a 15% increase in your daily calories until your body gets used to it and your metabolism adapts. Slowly, slowly, catchy monkey.

Bulking and cutting

The phases of bulking (putting on weight through a calorie surplus and training) and cutting (losing weight through a calorie deficit and training) are often cyclical. Certain sports follow these phases, generally if they are competing and there are weight categories, such as in different weightlifting strands, boxing and even horse racing. Other professional sportspeople, like footballers, will do a cut (and some might follow with a bulk) after a break from training – during their downtime, they'll relax the training and indulge more, and then need to quickly get back into shape before the next season starts. You'll often hear about it too in relation to bodybuilding, when doing a bulk phase in order to get bigger, stronger and put on more muscle. Pre-competition, they'll then go into a calorie-reduction cut phase to get back their six-packs – you lose muscle mass on a cut (ideally not too much) and so the abs will become more defined. Other disciplines like Strongmen/women are in a permanent bulk phase, forever trying to get bigger and, in turn, stronger.

If you are bulking, which is harder than it might sound, try to avoid 'dirty bulking', which is when you try to get the calories through eating junk food. You'll end up feeling crap if those kinds of food make up the majority of your intake. Try to choose a balance of unprocessed foods that are naturally high in protein, slow-release carbs and fat. These will give you the energy you need to train and also, if you do a cut phase afterwards, it won't be so hard. Meal prepping can help to ensure you get the calories you need, especially if you have a hectic pace of life.

I don't bother with cut phases and, in terms of bulking, I maintain the same calorie surplus. Although I weigh about 230lb, I'm naturally lean – left to its own devices, my body would be more like a runner's than a bodybuilder's. Even though I sound like a prize dickhead, complaining about this, I'd quite like to lose my six pack (but struggle to shift it) because having a big belly can be a great asset lifting heavy weights.

Training

For those of you whose weight is at a healthy level, where you don't need to lose any, but you want to have a more shredded physique, I'd advise you to stick to your current calorie intake. When you're following a training plan (mine or another), an intense workout should be enough to make your body shape more sculpted, without the need to combine it with a reduction in calories. If you then want to build more muscle, you'd increase your calories little by little. And when choosing your training, remember that while cardio burns calories, it won't be getting you a shredded aesthetic – if that's what you're after, incorporate some resistance training into your exercise regime. When you do this type of exercise you burn calories during and after the session, even while you rest, and you build muscle. And by the way, your calorie targets, whether surplus or deficit, should be the same on the days you don't exercise as the ones you do.

A note on calories if you're ever injured – if you're inactive, you'd want to avoid growing extra timber, but provided you're only out of action for a relatively short period of time, you might reduce calories but not drastically cut them unless you're intentionally trying to lose weight.

You do you

You might have heard people using the terms cutting, bulking, shredding etc. as if they were a badge of honour, things that should be aspired to. Sorry, but I really don't think anyone should be boasting about this, despite the endless #macrocounting, #ifitfitsyourmacros, #trackingmacros posts. Shouldn't we all just try to work hard and feel good without being too smug about it, boring the arse off people with how many or few calories they've had that day? I'm inviting you into the circle of trust as I tell you this secret: do what you want to do. If you truly feel well in yourself, then you don't need to cut or bulk. You should never be pressured into eating or exercising in a certain way in a bid to gain the respect of someone (either in 'real life' or in the weird world of online). It's up to you, so be happy in yourself.

Macros

You might have heard about tracking macros. Essentially this means you tot up the macronutrients in the food you're eating each day, ensuring you get the macronutrients you need and in the right ratio. This will vary per individual depending on the demands of their training. When you keep track of your macro targets every day, you will also be adding up your calorie intake at the same time. I think there's a balance to be found between being aware of what you're consuming without the need to be too evangelical about documenting every bite of apple you might have had. I'd suggest being mindful, but not getting too neurotic about it all. If you're making a big lifestyle change, keeping close track can be helpful, but you should soon find it becomes more intuitive and that you gravitate towards the foods your body needs.

If your diet doesn't support your workout, you'll make some gains, but not nearly as many as you could. For adaptation to take place, i.e. for your body to progress in exercise, you need adequate nutrition and good-quality rest (more on that in a bit).

Protein

Among its other superpowers, this essential macronutrient builds and repairs our body's tissues, helps create a strong immune system through the production of antibodies and is responsible for hormone production. When you are working out, particularly if you're doing strength training, you are deliberately damaging muscles in order for them to get stronger and grow – but this protein synthesis can only be sustained with adequate nutrition. If we don't get enough, it can lead to a catabolic state, when the muscle needs protein but there isn't enough there. When it comes to training, protein deficiency will cause muscle cramping, loss of muscle mass, lack of energy and general aches and pains, as our recovery from exercise takes longer. Protein intake is one of the first questions I ask fitness newbies about, and most of the time it's clear that they are lacking sufficient protein in their diet. It's easy to fall into the habit of meals being mainly carb-based: cereal for breakfast, sandwich for lunch and a bowl of pasta in the evenings. I'm all for carbs, but they need to be combined with other nutrients, not instead of them.

We all need protein in our diets, whether you're a lazy bollocks or if you're auditioning for world's strongest human, but the quantity varies depending on how active you are. As a general rule, a sedentary person requires 0.8g per kilo of body weight, whereas an active person needs around 2g per kilo (some people say that a little less, say 1.6g, is sufficient, but I like to advise the upper end). So, for me, as I'm around 110kg, my protein target is on the very high end of the spectrum, at around 220g per day. Now, I might not actually need that much, and I could probably maintain at around 190–200g per day, but I prefer to be certain I'm hitting my demands. It's particularly important to meet your protein requirements when you are exercising or trying to build muscle. Your body can only achieve so much if it doesn't have the right nutrition backing it – and protein is a major part of that. I am meticulous about ensuring I hit my protein goals each day, way more so than I am about counting calories. Get your laughing gear around some protein at every meal, spreading your intake over the course of the day rather than horsing it into you all in one go, at one mealtime. If you are training hard, try to consume around 25g protein (e.g. a small tin of tuna or a typical scoop of protein powder mixed into a smoothie) shortly after your workout. When following this approach with regards to what to eat when training, you'll hopefully find you eat a bit more intuitively. This is why I find I don't need to tot up my calories, because my body tells me when I need more and when I can stop.

I'm giving you this overview because knowing how it all affects the body will hopefully encourage you to be mindful about hitting your target each day – 'get it into ya, Cynthia' as they say in the States.

Protein is made up of around twenty amino acids, which are compounds that form the foundations of protein – nine essential (the ones we can't make ourselves and we need to get through food) and eleven non-essential (which the body naturally makes). Through our diets, we need to make sure we get these nine essential amino acids each day, and the easiest way to do this is through foods that contain a complete source of protein. 'Complete' refers to foods that have them all; animal products like eggs, fish and meat tend to be good for this, as well as some plant-based foods such as chia seeds and quinoa. Other plant-based foods have them too, but in an 'incomplete' way, meaning they have some but not all of these nine essential amino acids, so you need to eat a combination of foods such as lentils, veg and nuts to be reaching your amino acid needs each day.

The essential proteins that are found only in our diet are phenylalanine, valine, threonine, tryptophan, methionine, leucine, isoleucine, lysine and histidine. These all have properties better than fairy magic, and you need them all – hence the 'essential' part of their job title – but there are two I want to draw to your attention to in relation to training: leucine and isoleucine. Leucine, as well as making growth hormones and regulating blood sugar, is fundamental to muscle repair, while isoleucine is concentrated in muscle tissue and builds muscle metabolism. It also boosts immune function and regulates energy in the body.

It's not uncommon to be deficient in these essential amino acids, and you will notice the difference if you are training hard but not having enough of these in your diet. They can help prevent muscle breakdown, aid recovery post-workout and help improve overall strength. People often overlook the intricacies of their diet, especially when they're trying to figure out why they aren't making as much progress with exercise as they'd have thought. They naturally assume it's the training regime they're following and start playing around with that instead of uncovering a simpler explanation.

So, make sure you're getting dietary sources of these all-important amino acids by eating a variety of these foods throughout the day: milk, eggs, cheese, beef, pork, chicken, fish, nuts, seeds, soya beans, tofu, lentils, veg such as sweet potatoes, oats and wholegrains.

Now, back to non-essential amino acids – these are the eleven dudes your body makes by itself. Out of these, there are some that your body can only make if you move, including proline, glutamine and glycine. Are you sitting comfortably? Well you shouldn't be, because if so, you're not making them. Get out of your seat, you fecker, and read this book standing up!

Protein supplements

Your main source of protein should be from food, but depending on your target-number of grams per day, it can be a tall order getting it down the hatch. Protein supplements make up a part of my nutritional intake, by way of topping up what I get from food. Given my pretty high protein needs, it would be a big ask to get that from food alone (remember, 220g is equivalent to 30-odd eggs or 5 steaks each day!). Whey, which is derived from milk curds, is one of the most popular sources of protein that comes in powder form, making it easy to be stirred into things like smoothies, soups, pancake batter or your morning porridge. There are loads of vegan alternatives made from things like hemp, seeds and sprouted brown rice. *Mmm* – sounds yum.

Some people seem to be a bit apprehensive about the idea of supplementing with protein powder. They think it sounds unnatural or believe it might lead them to look like the Hulk just by drinking a protein shake every day. If only it were that easy to build muscle! In reality, adding some protein powder to your diet is sometimes just more convenient than griddling some sea bass before you leave for work in the morning. If you can reach your protein allowance through food alone, then hats off to you, but otherwise a powder is a safe option that is relatively low in calories and fairly inexpensive per 'portion'.

As I said, think food first, with supplements supporting your diet. These are obviously great for a high concentration of protein but they are very much lacking in the other essential nutrients needed for a healthy, strong body. There's been a big boom-time in the protein business and it can be confusing knowing which type to go for, and when it's best to consume protein. Here are a few to keep an eye out for:

Casein: This is a slow-release protein – I have this before bed to be released gradually overnight.

Whey protein isolate: This is a purer form of protein supplement, which hits straight away. Muscle protein synthesis occurs in the recovery period straight after training, so as soon as I do a workout I have whey protein isolate in a milkshake or smoothie.

Concentrate: Like isolate, this is a fast-hitting protein. As it's a concentrate, depending on the brand it might contain other ingredients like HMB (a leucine metabolite) or added vitamins and minerals – so read the ingredients list to make sure you're happy with what's in there.

Isoleucein: I always look out for this little fella because it boosts recovery in the muscles after a workout.

Creatine: Some protein supplements contain this. It regenerates your body's energy source, ATP, which will in turn boost your energy. (I have creatine coming out of my eyeballs; I've been mainlining it for the past decade.)

Other things to think about:

- Work out how much protein you need daily, depending on your body weight and training routine (an online calculator can help you determine this if you're not sure). A beginner or intermediate won't need as much protein as an elite because they aren't working so hard and tearing muscle tissue.
- If you are comparing brands for quality or price, check the amount of protein in the grams per serving, as these vary.

- Have a look at how your protein of choice has been manufactured, for example if it has been heat-treated or cold-pressed, or whether it is derived from organic milk (if you're using an animal-based product). These factors can have a big bearing on price too.
- If possible, try to buy in bulk, which will be more economical.
- Choose a taste and texture you like – you'll be gobbling it up at least once a day, so it's gotta be nice. Powders come in a variety or flavours, or you can just buy an unflavoured one which you can then add your own to, for example if you mix it with fruit or veg, nut butters or cocoa powder.

Here are the approximate amounts of protein in some everyday foods that are good sources.

ANIMAL SOURCES (PER 100G):

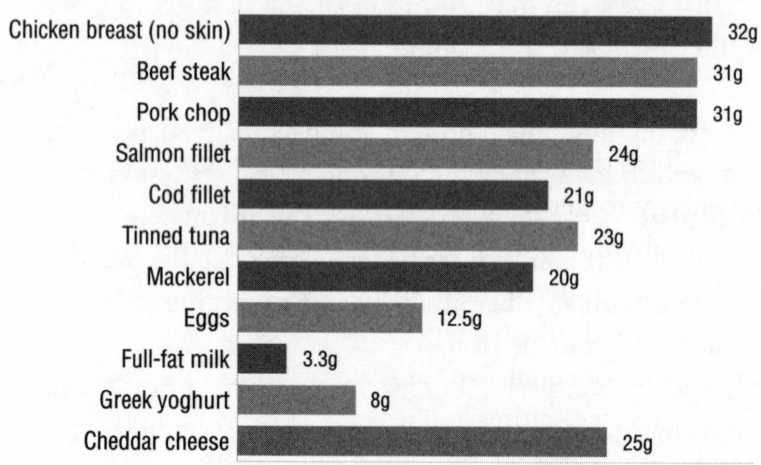

PLANT-BASED SOURCES (PER 100G):

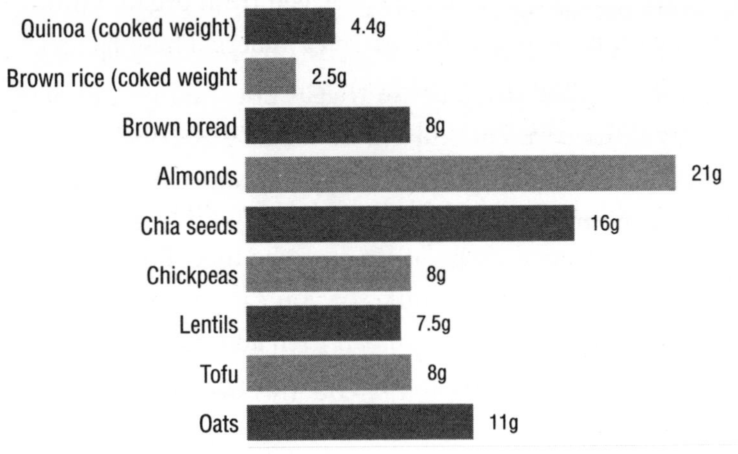

Carbohydrates

I've never met a carb I didn't like. This macronutrient is broken down into glucose, giving energy to the body, and fuelling brain and nerve cells. I often get asked about carbs, particularly by clients who might be following a calorie deficit – going carb-free is, to many, the 'secret' to losing weight. Carbs have been demonised, but they are an essential part of a balanced diet and I would never suggest cutting them out, especially as they are the very foods that are going to give you the energy to get to the gym in the first place!

'Carbohydrates' is a term that describes many different foods, from grains like wheat and oats, to fruit and veg and to processed foods like fizzy drinks, crisps and sweets, so they're very much not equal. Nutrient-dense complex carbohydrates like brown rice, pulses and leafy green veg will provide you with healthy carbs, along with other essential nutrients such as fibre, vitamins and minerals. If these types of unprocessed foods make up the bulk of your carb intake, it will help maximise your performance when exercising, not least because you'll be feeling well in yourself. The other magic trick carbs can perform is that any glucose that is not used by the body for energy is stored as back-up in the form of glycogen. This is the fuel that kicks in if you ever do a workout that has burned through all your available glucose.

Fats

Fats give our body energy, which are also stored as a back-up for times when we need a fuel injection. Fats support brain development and memory, and they also help to keep the nerves throughout the body in tip-top condition. The benefit that is most important to me, though, is that fats, such as omega-3, help keep the hair voluptuous.

Healthy fats are a vital part of an athlete's diet (and should be for mere mortals too). As with carbs, they've been given a bad rep in the past, so it's no wonder we're all a bit confused about these fellas. Doctors used to tell us that saturated fats (found more in animal-based foods) were 'bad' and unsaturated fats (found mostly in plant-based foods) were 'good', but with more research emerging, it seems that it's not as simple as we used to believe. The healthier fats I try to include in my diet come from good-quality red meat, oily fish, olive oil, nuts, seeds and avocado. I never go for low-fat products in the supermarket; for me it's full-fat milk all the way. I find full-fat tastes better and, while it is processed, it's often less processed and tends to have fewer additives that the lower-calorie equivalent – and, anyway, I need those calories! But for someone looking to cut calories, reducing the intake of fat-rich foods may be a good idea as they are the most calorie-dense macronutrient.

Like everything we eat, portion sizes when it comes to the fats we include in our diet should be regulated, and those on a calorie deficit should be particularly mindful of this.

The one thing everyone is in agreement about is watching our trans-fats intake. These can be found in packets of biscuits, cakes, pastries, sweets and margarine. If you see a product like this with a long best-before date, the chances are it contains trans-fats. And I can't lie to you, my beloved takeaways contain them, which is why they're not a daily occurrence. So keep trans-fats to a minimum (or avoid altogether).

REST AND RECOVERY

Giving your body time to heal and regenerate is an essential component of fitness, so you'll be pleased to hear that having a good kip will boost your sporting performance. And when you're injured or run-down, taking the time to recover properly is absolutely essential to coming back to exercise fighting fit.

Injury and recovery

> 'You start off your career hearing horror stories about long-term absences from the field, without ever thinking it'll happen to you. Having been on the receiving end of 13 months of injury, amid numerous other setbacks, taught me so much about what money can't buy.'
>
> ANTHONY WATSON, ENGLAND AND BATH RUGBY PLAYER

A pec torn off the bone, torn left tricep tendon, broken right wrist, chipped clavicle, fried SI joints, torn knee ligaments, broken right fibula, torn left ankle ligaments – these are just some of the knocks I've had over the years.

Injury is every athlete's worst nightmare, but pretty unavoidable. After moving from Esher to Old Elthamians, in pre-season training I got gang-tackled (where two people tackle, one above and one below) and it caused serious injury. I tore the tendons in my tricep, which is something that still plagues me to this day. I'd had various injuries before, but nothing like this. I didn't take the proper measures to allow myself to recover and I kept re-tearing it, both playing rugby and by lifting weights at the gym. I was far too impatient to be injured.

In some respects, I suppose injury ended up leading me to some other pretty great things; I do like to think that even the shittiest of circumstances can have a silver lining. During my rugby years, I started doing a bit of sports modelling. I was the face of Technogym's Pure Strength campaign (and you'll probably still see me on a lot of their machines around the world!), and worked with various companies on their PR campaigns. I stopped playing rugby not long after my tricep damage, and it was hard to make the finances work as it wasn't super-well paid. By being injured, I'd lost a job working with a big brand. It was a real blow to my finances and it made me question whether I should be playing rugby at all. I loved the game, but it was making me vulnerable to injury, which in turn was affecting my ability to earn a living.

Injury's crap. I don't want to sound too flippant, especially when injuries can range hugely in seriousness and have lasting damage, but if it strikes, you just have to get on with it, look after yourself as best you can and do what you can to try to prevent it recurring. If you are training at an intermediate or elite level, depending on your discipline, you can expect an injury to occur at some stage. For example, in my sport, powerlifting, 80% of people get injured twice a year. This doesn't necessarily mean you'll be benched while you're injured; it's just that you might have to adapt your training so you can continue to work out while you heal. A huge number of top-tier athletes are competing with some level of injury, minding themselves as they do so.

Always, always, ALWAYS get treatment and advice from a doctor and/or physio when you have an injury. Don't be a hero and ignore niggles, because they could lead to something far worse. Remember, too, that your body is a clever sod, and so when something isn't feeling quite right, it might be because your technique needs improving. Sometimes a simple adjustment will not only make you feel loads better, it'll massively improve your performance too.

Remember that after an injury has improved or recovered totally, with any swelling or pain having subsided, there might be an imbalance around it because the joint, muscle, bone or whatever will have been out of action for a while. Resist the urge to go back to balls-to-the-walls training and make sure you talk to a physio about rectifying and strengthening these imbalances.

Sometimes you have to make tough decisions about treating injuries. It's painful watching top sportspeople having to drop out of tournaments they'd probably win because the strenuous effort of going for gold might cause serious damage to their body. All that training and mental preparation, only to be derailed at the eleventh hour. When I tore my tricep tendon off, I should have had surgery to reattach it and to recover properly, but I didn't want to pause my training. I now can't lock out my left arm. Should I have taken time out to let my body recover? Most likely. It feels hard to stop, though, especially when you love the sport you do and have goals you're trying to reach. The frustration makes you just want to get back out there. Having a positive mindset – as with every part of life! – helps when dealing with an injury, so you can focus on the steps you can take to get back out there, like getting expert advice, doing mobility exercise and other rehab. Thankfully, I now know more about how to avoid more easily preventable injuries, and one major way is through mobility (see page 177 for a reminder).

But it's not all doom and gloom, folks. Many athletes overcome setbacks and return stronger and fitter than ever. Look at Serena Williams, who played some of her best ever tennis less than a year after complicated childbirth left her bed-bound for six weeks.

Recovery between training sessions

The time it takes to recover will depend on the type of training you're doing as well as how often you're doing it. There are some other factors too, such as age and general wellbeing, including how much sleep you're getting and overall nutrition (particularly if you're not hitting nutritional components such as adequate protein intake). How you are feeling in yourself generally can impact recovery – for example, if you're under the weather, have any injuries or are suffering from stress. It's not always easy to strike the balance, and in the past when, quite frankly, I didn't really know what I was doing, I often failed to give myself proper time to recover. Exercise can put a massive strain on our bodies; they can't tolerate constantly working out. Our bodies interpret exercise as a form of stress, so it's important to be mindful of this. It can be extra hard to allow yourself to rest if you feel that not being in the gym or out exercising is hampering your progress, slowing down your goals. But actually the reverse is true. You will only safely reach your targets if you allow yourself to properly recover. I know I will only be able to reach my next target by scheduling rest days in my workouts, and it's a non-negotiable for me now. So, reframe these rest days as helping you get closer to your targets, not moving away from them.

Sleep

We're supposed to spend one third of our lives doing it, but lack of sleep must be one of the great tragedies of our time! And I do believe the old saying is true, that things look rosier in the morning – but IMO that's only after a good night's kip. It can't be a coincidence that as we spend more time on our phones, the less sleep we seem to get. Insomnia is on the up, either with people finding they take longer to get to sleep or they wake up in the night – or even a bit of both, for some poor feckers. Sleep is always a big focus for professional athletes, and many of them even receive a specially tailored plan so that they maximise their rest to support body and mind. Imagine Paralympian sprinter Jonnie Peacock trying to compete for a gold medal after tossing and turning the night before – I wouldn't fancy his chances. Nothing will improve your performance more significantly than decent sleep – no supplement, no special piece of equipment, no PT – and here's why:

Strength: Catching forty winks is even more important when you're exercising, and that's because training puts demands on the body, including muscle and tissue damage, and it's through rest that they get a chance to rebuild. Sleep helps your body's cells repair and allows you to recover from your workouts faster, helping you build strength.

Physical maintenance: Sleeping protects your central nervous system, helps consolidate memories, lowers your heart rate, triggers the release of waste products from your organs and reduces inflammation in the body. In *Why We Sleep*, neuroscientist Matthew Walker explains how sleep boosts your whole physical wellbeing by helping to reduce the likelihood of suffering from conditions such as heart disease, type 2 diabetes and obesity.

Appetite: Lack of sleep can slow down the metabolism, whereas good rest encourages hormone balance, helping to regulate appetite by not interfering with your hunger signals (i.e. making you think your body is hungry when it's actually not, which can cause over-eating). You might also find that when you feel knackered, you need to eat more – and often we gravitate towards sugar-rich treats for that instant energy burst, just to help us stay alert, which can lead to weight gain and other health problems if you're not expending the calories through exercise.

Mental wellbeing: I hope you never meet me after I've been awake half the night thanks to my sleep-stealing toddler, because I am like the antichrist. Sleep deprivation massively affects our mood, leaving us irritable, slower to complete tasks, unfocused and stressed. Sleep disorders lead to an increase in car accidents and tend to make sufferers more accident-prone in general. A chronic sleep deficit can (very understandably) result in low mood, depression and anxiety, and there's a bit of a catch-22 going on here because, if you suffer from those conditions in the first place, they might be keeping you awake.

Just as sleep helps to motivate you to exercise and enhances your performance when you do, exercise also aids sleep. In Part 1 we looked at all the ways movement benefits our mental health, lowering stress and releasing feel-good chemicals into the body, putting us in fine fettle. Stress, depression and anxiety, however, are big barriers to sleep.

Revive: Waking up feeling rested is far more likely to lead to your daily constitutional, whereas it's a big ask to get your rear in gear and out to exercise if you wake up feeling wrecked. And when you do get out there when you feel restored, your performance, endurance and stamina will be better – and you'll enjoy it more!

The whys and hows of sleep

The World Health Organization recommends we get eight hours of sleep a night – the ideal amount varies per individual, but most of us thrive on somewhere between seven to nine hours. And depending on how much physical activity you're doing, you'll likely need to achieve the higher end of the scale. And it's not just quantity – the quality can't be overlooked, either, so if you're getting eight hours a night but rousing during that period, then that's probably not enough. You go through various stages of REM and non-REM sleep each night, with brain activity changing depending on the stage you're in. These stages serve different functions in the body, but if you're not managing to reach the deep phase of sleep each night or not spending long enough there, then you won't feel rested and restored the next day.

If you're a lark, you'll naturally head to bed relatively early, wake up the next day without needing to set an alarm and be in good spirits in the mornings. If, though, you feel more energised in the evenings and prefer staying up later, and a sledgehammer knocking through your gaff won't rouse you in the mornings, then you're an owl. And it's pretty common to be a bit of both (hands up if you like a lie-in *and* an early night). The world tends to be tailored to chirpy larks – having to get up at the crack of dawn to get to work or school is hard-going for an owl. If you've any choice in the matter, play to your strengths by following your circadian rhythms and fitting work and fun around the times you have the most stamina.

Slumber hormones and nutrients

Our hormones can help make or break our quality of sleep, so here are some ways to get our body's chemicals on side, including utilising some secret food weapons you may be overlooking. These can trigger sleep-boosting hormones, because they contain amino acids which help us to wind down. And there are some key minerals in the body that will naturally encourage zonking out . . .

Serotonin is a brain chemical created during sleep which passes messages between cells and plays a vital role in regulating our mood. Sleep deprivation lowers the amount of serotonin in the body, and can cause or exacerbate feeling low. One of the best ways to trigger the release of serotonin is through exercise.

Melatonin is one of the big daddies of chemicals, as it helps regulate the production of other chemicals in the body. It's also responsible for your sleep cycles, letting your body know when to wake and rest. Melatonin has been manufactured into pill form, which is sometimes prescribed by doctors to help treat insomnia, but to get a natural kick, include oats, tomatoes, sweetcorn, cherries, peanuts and sunflower seeds in your diet.

Tryptophan is an amino acid and antioxidant which is needed to produce the neurotransmitter serotonin, which helps regulate sleep and balance mood. Milk, yoghurt, poultry and pumpkin seeds are good natural sources.

Magnesium is an essential nutrient that does various maintenance in the body including helping to keep your heart rhythm and blood pressure in good nick. It also helps in the development of bone and regulates muscle contraction and nerve function. Working alongside its pal serotonin, it can also help you relax, because it calms your nervous system. Cashew nuts, almonds, spinach, soya milk, brown rice and potatoes are good sources, and it's also sometimes added to foods like breakfast cereal.

Low levels of **vitamin D** have been linked with various sleep disorders, as this can affect sleep and wake cycles, seriously damaging the overall quality of your sleep. You can get vitamin D through your diet by eating foods such as eggs, salmon, sardines, mushrooms (leave them under a window to pimp their vitamin D content rather than storing in the fridge) and certain fortified breakfast cereals, and also through sunlight. Because the UK isn't blessed with a lot of sunshine, Public Health England recommends that people consider taking a vitamin D supplement of 10mcg, especially during autumn and winter, because it's tricky getting it from food alone.

Potassium and **calcium** are minerals that can help with relaxation as well as maintaining healthy blood sugar levels – both of which can aid deeper sleep. Potassium is an electrolyte that supports muscle growth, heart function and nerve reflexes in the body, and it's thought that it can encourage fewer disturbances, such as muscle spasms, through the night once you get to sleep. Bananas, sweet potatoes, broccoli, black beans and dried fruit like raisins and dates are all good sources. Calcium helps the brain produce melatonin, and if you were paying attention a few minutes ago you'll know this regulates sleep cycles – so there's likely some truth in the age-old sleep hack of having a cup of hot milk before bed. As well as dairy products, calcium is found in hazelnuts, sardines and kale. If you want to combine calcium and potassium in one fell swoop, you could whip up a smoothie of milk or yoghurt with a banana, half an avocado and a date or two.

Now we know which hormones are beneficial to sleep, here are some chaps you want to keep at bay when you're trying to bunk down. Your stress hormones **adrenaline** and **cortisol** rise when the body feels it needs to switch to survival mode. They tend to speed up mental activity, often making your thoughts race. They can also cause a physical response in the body, like a racing heart, sweating, twitching or needing to pace around – the enemies of a relaxed sleep!

Watch what you eat and drink

So, having a balanced diet, which includes enough of the foods just mentioned, should be part of your everyday routine. And here are a few things to remember, especially if good sleep is escaping you.

- **Caffeine**, which is in coffee, tea, fizzy drinks, chocolate, and even some medicines, like those flu remedies, affects everyone differently. Some people can drink coffee all evening and have no trouble sleeping soundly all night, but this isn't the case with many others. If you're not sure of your tolerance to its side effects, just err on the side of caution and avoid it altogether for at least eight hours before bedtime, i.e. if you're hitting the sack at 10 p.m. your last mug of builder's should be no later than 2 p.m. (I know you'll probably still be hitting it at 4 p.m. as you try to power through the afternoon, so do what you want – just remember it might come back to bite you in the arse later on.)
- Keep well **hydrated** during the day so that you don't wake up in the night thirsty. Drinking around about 2 litres of water per day will stop you stirring in the night because you are parched.
- **Booze** can make you drowsy, especially if you're hitting it hard, but it will definitely disturb your sleep quality. Again, its effects vary from person to person – some find that a glass or two of wine makes no difference, whereas others will notice that even one beer will get in the way of a sound night's sleep. The problem is that, even if you drop off quickly, if you've hit the sauce you're much more likely to wake up throughout the night – fidgeting, needing a slash, being dehydrated and getting hot and bothered – and you won't enter the long, restful, deep phase of sleep. For me, though,

from time to time a night on the tiles is worth missing a night's sleep for!

- **Smoking** and **vaping**: there's no point in me giving you an ear-bashing if you're a smoker, but I will say here that smoking before bed can cause problems dropping off and can keep a person in the lighter, less restorative phases of sleep. Nicotine is a stimulant and can bring alertness both to your mind and also your body, as your heart speeds up. This might be one of the reasons that, overall, smokers seem to get less sleep than non-smokers.
- Eating shortly before bedtime, as well as snaffling **foods that are high in sugar or very processed,** can lead to indigestion as the gut tries to break down the little 'gift' you've just given it. It can also disrupt blood sugar levels, meaning you might be more likely to wake up again once you have dropped off.
- Varied grub that includes all the **macro- and micro-nutrients** will help lull you to sleep. Diets that lack key nutrients, like those that follow protein-heavy plans which leave out wholesome carbs, often cause individuals to wake up more at night. Similarly, going to bed feeling really hungry isn't a great idea, as it'll lead to you rouse more in the night, with your belly wondering where its next snack is.

Top tips for good kips

We know that our sleep habits affect the quality and duration of our rest. The most important thing to do to get a quality night's sleep is to get rid of your children, if you have any.

Preferably sell them in a bid to make a small return on the shitload of shoes, nappies, Lego etc. you've invested in them so far. I won't go into the science of this equation (too complicated and you'll be too tired to understand) but essentially: sleep + kids = ☹. If, unfortunately, you are not able to find a buyer for them, here are some other rules for lights out. I'd like to say I do these every night, but let's just say here are all the things I (am trying to) do.

During the day

- As soon as you get out of bed, open any curtains or blinds throughout your home – the natural light will send an immediate signal to your body clock that it's go-time.
- Next on the list is – drum roll . . . exercise. Of course it is. Being active is one of the best ways you can boost your serotonin levels, which helps lull you to sleep. As we know, it can also help reduce stress and anxiety, leaving you less likely to struggle to get to sleep as you stare at the ceiling.
- If you're partial to a catnap, particularly if you've slept badly the night before, go for it – be sure it's no longer than 20 minutes, though, as after this you enter a deeper phase of sleep.
- Limit technology: I know we've all heard this before and I am awful for staring at my phone lying in bed. Not only can it stress us out (sometimes unknowingly) looking at our newsfeed, scrolling through social media or assessing our to-do list/calendar of doom, but the blue light that emerges from our tech can really impact on our sleep.

Have a wind-down routine

You have to tell your body it's time to prepare for sleep so that it knows to transition to that mode. Very few people can go from being fully active and 'on' to dropping asleep at the drop of a hat. Just as they do for kids, routines can help alert our brain that wakey-wakey time is coming to an end.

- Try to keep evenings calm so that you have plenty of time to relax before hitting the hay. Going to bed at the same time every evening will help your biological clock fall into a predictable rhythm.
- Keep lights dim in the evening, using lamps instead of overhead lights where possible, to help unwind.
- Try to avoid getting worked up in the evenings – this sometimes happens without us consciously noticing it. Checking emails or even watching something on TV like a thriller or an action film, or reading an exciting book, can increase our stress levels and take longer to come down from.
- Having a bath or shower shortly before bed will signal to your body that sleep is on its way. When your body's temperature gradually cools after being risen in a bath or shower, your body realises it's heading towards night-time mode and an urge to sleep should kick in.

Your sleep space

- It's amazing how much money we spend on other areas of our lives, such as clothes, eating out and taking trips, yet loads of us sleep on ratty old mattresses, limp pillows and bed sheets that look like someone might have died on them. I reckon you should all treat yourself to the best you can afford, and at the very least replace your pillows every two or three years (those sad, floppy ones can cause neck ache too).

- Set up your sleep environment. Open your bedroom window as you get ready for bed, giving the room a blast of fresh air. Keep all overhead lights off, making the room as dim as possible – signalling to your brain that sleep is around the corner. Clear up any clutter in your bedroom before bedtime, as it's hard to unwind if you're looking at your jocks on the floor.
- Use your bed for sleep and sex. Nigella Lawson apparently keeps ketchup and mustard next to her bed, ready to devour a freshly made culinary treat while sitting up in bed in one of her famous silky dressing gowns. But then she's the nation's favourite domestic goddess and you're not – the rules are different for Nigella. So, for mere mortals like us, no eating, no working on your laptop, no watching telly.
- I can't pretend I'm a great man for scented candles or essential oils, but many people find the aromas relaxing.

If you can't get to sleep

- Trying not to worry too much about sleep can help take the pressure off *getting* to sleep. And yeah, I get it – as soon as someone tells you to stop worrying about X, it's all you can think about. If your brain is spinning on its axis, try to slow it down by scribbling down in a notebook, kept by the bed, any worries or to-dos. You might feel a bit more relaxed once you put them on paper, ready to sort out the following day.

- Don't check the time or look at your phone! Seeing how long you've been lying down waiting for sleep to come is really stressful, especially if you then do the maths on how few hours you might potentially get before the alarm goes off in the morning.
- This is a good trick to release physical tension, especially if you've been exercising during the day. Focus on every area of your body in turn, starting from your feet, going up to your ankles, legs and up through the body, finishing with your head. Tense each body part for a few seconds and then release. Think of all the work each bit has done that day as it supported you – give all your bones and joints a little TTFN (ta ta for now!).
- If your sleep problems go on for longer than a few weeks, don't suffer in silence – check in with your GP.

GO THE DISTANCE

If you've made it to here, you've got further than I have with 99.9% of the books I've ever started, and you might be glad to hear we're almost at the finish line. I wanted to round up with a few last witterings to launch you on your way.

Confidence and motivation: I talked a lot about these at the start of the book and we're coming full circle, back to the source. If there are only a couple of things you take away from this book, make it these. Not how to deadlift or reach your running PB. Not how much protein you need to scoff or how the cardiovascular system works. Confidence and motivation. If you have one, you'll have the other, and likewise if one is missing the other will plummet. These will go up and down throughout life, soaring sky-high when something goes your way – for example, when that promotion at work boosts your confidence and motivates you to slog away twice as hard. Or, on the flip side, your boss says something out of order and you lose all incentive to work hard. But confidence and motivation are the secret to achieving the life you want, full of meaningful stuff: good relationships with people who are kind, who make you laugh and who respect you (behind all the banter), as well as striving to make tomorrow a teeny bit better than today. Confidence and motivation – these are your true north.

Think about the power of intention – it's all well and good to come up with an idea but until you step into that intention, get up and actually do it, it's just a pipe dream. Intention is a powerful energy that I find really motivates me. It's up to you, not anyone else, to make what you want happen. Hold yourself accountable and keep your standards for yourself high. If you have a niggling feeling you truly should be doing a different job, going out with someone else or taking care of your body better, follow your instinct and do it, but separate your true gut feeling from any noise and chatter. Once you start being kinder to your body, making more mindful choices about your health, you'll find it much easier to tap into intuition. Everything you need is within you, and homing into the magic of positive thinking will bring you the mental fortitude of Arya Stark (tell me you've seen *Game of Thrones*? If not, you're dead to me). Fostering a cheerier outlook (even if you were born a miserable git) will help you get fit, stay fit or push your boundaries of fitness. Where the mind leads, the body will follow.

I told you earlier in the book that how I look doesn't motivate me in the slightest; I just don't care about aesthetics. So, if I'm ever in need of motivation, it's not from the thought of seeing a six-pack in the mirror but from thinking of how I am reaching my lifting goals and also how my workouts are supporting my wider health. As Harvard paleoanthropologist Daniel Lieberman says, 150 minutes of moderate physical activity a week can help prolong your life. It's hard to argue with that. The other reason I rarely miss a workout is that I'd be climbing up the walls if I didn't. I don't sleep well if I haven't burnt off some energy and I miss those endorphins.

Life will sometimes get in the way (Oh hiya, global pandemic) – not to worry because when you have to pause or when you encounter a setback, it's always possible to get back on the wagon and recalibrate your goals. You know how to do that now and it's made easier when you think about the journey as much as the results. I feel like a wise old sage spouting out all this, so please imagine me wearing some red robes in bare feet, wandering round a garden occasionally ringing a bell or talking to a bird (instead of wearing trackies, drinking a protein shake and furiously bashing away at my keyboard).

Screw it, let's do it

Micro-changes is a slightly irritating buzzword that's been doing the rounds for ages, but I do think there's something in it, especially when it comes to improving wellbeing. Have you ever watched the Marie Kondo series where she tries to help people throw their junk away? So, she goes into the homes of... I'm trying to think of a polite word for these... collectors – I know, let's call them *maximalists.* In some of their homes, you can barely get through the front door, they have so much stuff. It's chaos, but don't worry, Marie's going to sort them out. In she comes with a slightly manic glint in her eye, and she always starts the same way – tackling just one space at a time. For example, she'll hop like a sprite into the bedroom and throw everything out of the wardrobe with wild abandon. Literally rifling through people's drawers. She piles up clothes onto the bed and you can see all her Christmases have come at once as she asks the poor chump (who can't resist a sale, if the eighteen blue t-shirts are anything to go by) to separate the wheat from the chaff. Never – ever – does Queen Marie tackle more than one space at a time; one room is always completed before moving on to the next. Otherwise it would be carnage in the kitchen, lunacy in the lounge, disarray in the dining room (I'll stop now) all at once, and the homeowner would give it great guns at the start, only to lose momentum and give up, finding themselves in an even worse state than when they started out. Instead they nail the bedroom and, full of confidence, building on that success, they're ready for the sitting room. Now, that's good telly. *For the love of God, he's not going to try to make us fold our pants, is he? Where is he going with this?!* you cry.

Well, I reckon Marie is on to something, because the same approach goes for big lifestyle overhauls. I'm all for a resolution to live better, but as we looked at in Part 1, start small and don't throw the babba out with the bath water. You wake up one summer morning and decide, 'Right, I'm going away in four weeks and need to be bikini-ready, so nothing more than a lettuce leaf will pass my lips until then. And, while I'm at it, I'm going to get two gym memberships, a class pass and a personal trainer, and I'm going to work out all day, every day. And for good measure I'm going to pack in my 9–5, throw away the TV and cancel all my plans until 2031, so that I can completely focus on my health and fitness aspirations.' Come on now, let's not be silly. Unless you are in the extreme minority of people who can make a radical life-transformation work, then smaller steps are far more sustainable, making you much more likely to stick with it and get to where you want to be.

I'm telling you now, there aren't any shortcuts to true fitness, and neither should there be. It is about hard graft, putting in the time and making lasting changes to boost your health. But when you start by making smaller changes in your life, they often lead to much bigger and much needed alterations. Consistency is key to progression, and it's this that enables us to push ourselves beyond our comfort zone. Sounds a bit boring put like that, doesn't it? Here you were, thinking it must all be about being a mad bastard. Not the case, I'm afraid.

In Part 1, I wrote about a few theories that have struck a chord with me, and now here's another one – a little nugget I wanted to save for the end. The term 'marginal gains' is one you might have heard before. It's all about how little changes we make in our lives can all add up to significant improvement. It's not about a big-ass, scary life-transformation but tiny changes that build up to become more than the sum of their parts. Sir David Brailsford was the performance director leading Team GB to an incredible seven-gold-medal win for track cycling at the Beijing Olympics. (Nice job, Dave.) His thinking in the pre-Olympic training strategy was to break down everything that goes into riding a bike, including peripheral, often forgotten stuff like the kit used and the mattresses the cyclists slept on at night, which would maximise their sleep. Every tiny element was put under the microscope with the aim that if you can make an improvement of just 1% across many areas, they'll add up to a significant gain overall. It's a strategy that has been embraced in all walks of life, from sports to business.

What if you applied marginal gains theory to support your workouts? It might look something like this:

- Invest in sportswear that you love and feel good wearing. It doesn't have to be expensive – there are loads of brands making lower-cost options.
- Always have your clean kit or equipment ready to go in a bag, waiting for when it's next needed. It's not very motivating fishing a manky pair of shorts out of the laundry basket (trust me, I know).
- Pre-book any fitness classes or reserve any pitches or courts depending on what you're playing.
- Make time in your calendar in advance so that you make exercise happen.
- Get enough sleep to give you the energy to work out.
- Stock up on good-quality, fresh food at home, including high-protein snacks, so that you can have a diet that supports your exercise of choice.
- Don't worry, be happy. Easier said than done, but stress takes its toll on body and mind, preventing you from getting out to exercise (which is the very thing that might help).

So, *do* sweat the small stuff – it's the nitty-gritty that will see you through.

Always learning

Full disclosure: when I started as a PT, I made all kinds of mistakes. And no doubt there's advice I give in this book which may, in a few years, become out of date. We can only go on what we know now, keeping as informed as possible with new theories or evidence that emerges, and be willing to say, 'Oh, I got that one wrong.' This happens all the time in fields like medicine and public health – it's not that long ago that you'd go into a bar or restaurant only to be greeted by a cloud of smoke, as everyone was puffing away on fags indoors. And it wasn't *that* long ago (relatively speaking!) that people believed the Earth was flat, and there's so much out there we're still trying to understand (black holes, dark energy – what's it all about?!). We're learning all the time as new evidence changes our understanding. And remember, it's our old mucker confidence again that enables someone to say, 'I was misinformed there,' or even 'I don't know the answer to that Q.' There's still so much we don't know about the body, about fitness, about our health, but clinging to old advice and being too arrogant to admit mistakes is a mug's game. We just have to do the best we can with the info we've got. So, let's not be afraid to get it wrong or to fail – these can be great motivators, as you'll want to do better next time.

GAME, SET AND MATCH

'Nurture your roots and your flowers will bloom.'

PROVERB

'Do the small stuff and your beast will unleash.'

BLACK ZEUS

Can you imagine what would happen if everyone in this country gave up 30 minutes of screen time each day and started exercising instead? I can't help thinking of the bigger picture there. Maybe it would mean that obesity rates would decline (currently one in four of us is obese) and correlated conditions such as high blood pressure and heart disease (among many others) would fall. In turn, would we feel more energetic? Would kids be better able to concentrate in school? Would we meet more people by going to gyms and playing team sports and be more connected to our community? Would we relieve some pressure on local services and the NHS, with the effects of exercise helping to stave off some everyday illnesses as well as chronic ones? Would our mental health flourish from our bodies feeling that bit better and from the surge of stress-busting happy hormones from doing everyday tasks with ease and by spending the time normally devoted to looking at a screen doing something physical instead? It doesn't seem unrealistic that fitness could make the world a better place.

There's a theory in medicine that any mental or physical conditions we face are down to three things: our biology, psychology and sociology. Whether or not we enjoy good health comes down to a combination of factors – some we might have little control over, but many we do.

Symptoms of preventable physical ill health can often be traced back to lack of good mental wellbeing, and the same applies the other way round. Heart disease, obesity and depression are among the biggest killers of the global population. Mental health conditions such as depression can be complicated and occur for all sorts of reasons and I'm not saying exercise is a magic bullet that will cure all ills, but I do think that, for some people, it could help manage or ease symptoms.

So, if you've hit upon things that might have been holding you back, then I hope you find some inspiration to move beyond them or seek support wherever you can – asking for help is always a sign of strength, not weakness. Life is full-on. We bang on so much about the 'what next' that we can sometimes skip over the 'now'. Feeling like we need to be 'achieving' all the time can come at the expense of our day-to-day enjoyment of life's small things (the joy of cold pizza for breakfast, anyone?). There's a law of attrition there which can grind us down. While I do encourage having goals (big or small) to work towards, what I would love you to take away is to enjoy the process of exercise, rather than viewing it as box to tick off your to-do list.

I really hope you have discovered something in this book that motivates you to get up off the sofa and to move, or to push it to the next level, flying past your comfort zone to get fitter and more powerful that you ever imagined. A book has limitations, of course, and there are hundreds of fantastic ways to be fit; the few I've mentioned here are things that have worked for me, but the world is your oyster. Never before have there been so many ways to dip your toe in the water, with just about every type of fitness class available to glimpse or trial online, and often free of charge. Exercise shouldn't be a punishment – I promise you there'll be something out there you'll enjoy. Kayaking, pole vaulting or twerking – it all counts, so try some weird and wonderful activities until you hit the nail on the head.

You owe it to yourself to feel well every single day and to do everything within your power to future-proof your health – exercise is one of the very best ways to do that. Remember that, every time your children or kids in your neighbourhood see you out moving, you have normalised the practice of exercise. It's not a fad or quick fix; it's something to incorporate into your day-to-day for ever. At first that might seem daunting and unrealistic, but once you find something you love (and this may well chop and change – just go with it), before you know it it'll become a non-negotiable you won't need to 'make time for'; it'll be default. It shouldn't be something that some people do and others don't; it shouldn't depend on you age or your income; it should be universal.

So, a final brain-dump from me of things that I try to remember when I want to keep on keeping on:

- Be your unapologetic self.
- Don't take yourself too seriously. Take the piss and allow the same back (it's good to have a dose of our own medicine).
- It's quality over quantity: one legend of a friend, who gets you, warts and all, is better than ten

energy-drainers. Ditch any dweebs bringing you down and anyone who doesn't have your best interests at heart. Remember, snitches get stitches.

- Have a hug – studies have shown that having a hug lasting anywhere from 3 to 20 seconds can reduce stress (provided it's from someone you want to be hugged by!) by releasing happy, lovey hormones.
- You're not going to get it right all the time. It'd be weird if you did – you're not a robot – so accept that life is about learning on the job. Remember that optimists shrug off mistakes as an opportunity to grow; pessimists dwell on them, beating themselves up. Don't be one of those dudes; they're boring and no one wants to be around them. Whining is for wieners.
- Do something for others. It's not all about you. Donate to your local food bank or help a friend whenever you can. And, selfishly, it'll give you a warm, fuzzy feeling.
- Always wear denim with denim.*
- We can't expect to be deliriously euphoric every second of the day but you need to feel more than just *meh*. Aim high and remember life's great things are within your reach.
- Say thanks – to yourself, your god, the universe, whoever floats your spiritual boat. It doesn't have to be as vom-inducing as #blessed (I actually just did a little sick in my mouth there), but be grateful for the good things that happen each day. Doing this has been shown to make people more positive.

---

* Just seeing if you're awake. Obviously don't do double denim – it's a crime against humanity.

So, lads and lassies, there you have it. Now, remember: with great power comes great responsibility. You have the tools to do yourself proud. You're unstoppable, a force of nature, so believe in yourself (but not so much that you turn into a prat). Let exercise be for all of us. Here's to the underdogs (which we all are at various times in our life), the eccentrics, misfits and oddballs – there's room for all of us on the adventure to fitness.

REFERENCES

General reading

Crabbe, Tony, *Busy@Home* (Piatkus, 2020)
Duhigg, Charles, *The Power of Habit* (Random House, 2012)
Dwerk, Carol, *Mindset: Changing the Way You Think to Fulfil Your Potential* (Robinson, 2017)
Gale, Hazel, *The Mind Monster Solution* (Yellow Kite, 2019)
Jones, Kim, *222 Ways to Trick Yourself to Sleep* (Piatkus, 2019)
Kane, Owen, *Ten Times Happier* (HQ, 2020)
McRaven, Admiral William H., *Make Your Bed* (Michael Joseph, 2017)
Syed, Matthew, *Bounce: The Myth of Talent and the Power of Practice* (Fourth Estate, 2011)
Tracy, Brian, *Eat that Frog!* (Hodder, 2013)
Walker, Matthew, *Why We Sleep* (Penguin, 2018)
Wallace, Dr Hazel, *The Food Medic* (Yellow Kite, 2016)

Introduction

Dr John Ratey on All Hail Kale – Is Exercise Insanity?
www.allhailkale.com/podcasts-all-posts/is-exercise-insanity

Whole-body health

Prof. Daniel Lieberman on All Hail Kale – Is Exercise Insanity?
www.allhailkale.com/podcasts-all-posts/is-exercise-insanity

Energy systems

Training for Climbing Episode 21: energy system training
www.trainingforclimbing.com/podcast-21-energy-system-training-part-1/

Find your thing

Smart Consumer: Your Guide to the Fitness and Wellness Trends for 2020
www.bbc.co.uk/programmes/p07yhbxk

Wolf or bear?

www.futurelearn.com/courses/musculoskeletal/0/steps/25159

Plyometrics

www.frontiersin.org/articles/10.3389/fphys.2019.00178/full
www.ncbi.nlm.nih.gov/pmc/articles/PMC4637913/

mTOR pathway

Journal of Cell Science: jcs.biologists.org/content/122/20/3589

CHEERS

I'd like to say a heartfelt thank you to the following people and companies that have been instrumental in making this book happen.

Dan Parker aka Jerry Maguire and all the team at 84 World. Thank you for your constant belief and support. What a ride together so far and long may it continue.

Fritha Saunders and Kaiya Shang at Simon & Schuster: you have made a dream of mine come true and I will be forever grateful to you.

Genevieve Barratt and Harriet Collins: the dream team at Simon & Schuster. Thank you for all your hard work and ideas, and for ensuring that this is actually happening!

Simon & Schuster: 2020 has been such a strange year and I'm so sorry we haven't been able to all meet at your offices; however, please know that I massively appreciate all of the work you do behind the scenes, and I look forward to hugging you all in person soon!

Tamsin English: we hit it off in our very first meeting at Dean Street Townhouse, and knowing that I would have a fellow Irish person, with a great sense of humour, beside me to guide me and get what I am thinking down on paper with correct grammar has been amazing. You are truly a legend.

Oh and me for being me . . . also my mum for making me! 🖤🙌

INDEX

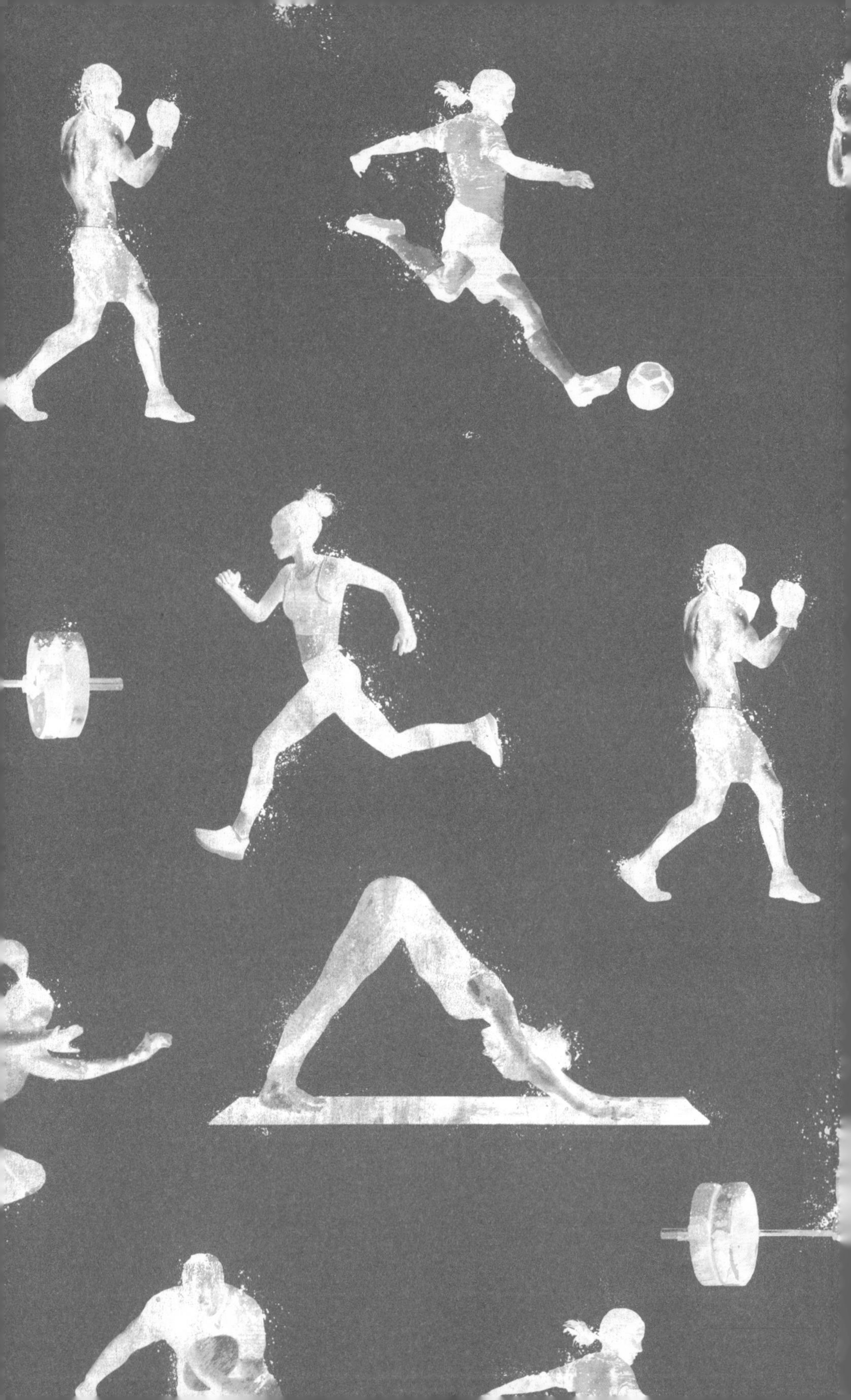